The
Remedy

The Five-Week Power Plan to Detox Your System, Combat the Fat, and Rebuild Your Mind and Body

Supa Nova Slom

HIP HOP'S MEDICINE MAN

WELLNESS CENTRAL

NEW YORK   BOSTON

Copyright © 2010 by Daoud Taheid Torain

Wellness Central
Hachette Book Group
237 Park Avenue
New York, NY 10017

www.HachetteBookGroup.com

Wellness Central is an imprint of Grand Central Publishing.
The Wellness Central name and logo are trademarks of Hachette Book Group, Inc.

Printed in the United States of America

First Edition: April 2010
10 9 8 7 6 5 4 3 2 1

Library of Congress Control Number: 2009933228

ISBN 978-0-446-56322-2

Contents

Note from Dr. Bernadette L. Sheridan

"And how are the children?"

In many cultures around the world, this sentence is a standard and customary greeting as a nation's wealth and prosperity is in direct proportion to the health of its youth. Sadly to say, as one who observes, chronicles, and is in the direct business of health and wellness, I can tell you that the most prosperous nation on planet Earth is in frightening contrast to the health of its most valuable asset: its youth. Statistically, it is an irrefutable fact that we are losing ground in many arenas of health. Things that used to manifest in older adults have now appeared in the hip-hop generation with a vengeance. Diabetes, hypertension, heart disease, and a host of other disorders are now the reality that links children with their parents. This is a disturbing, and even shameful, legacy.

America's future, our youth, also speak a different language. In their vernacular, their musical expression, it would appear that they have learned to cope with their parents' legacy by tuning them out in many ways. In order to heal and help them, it is imperative that we *connect* with them. What is needed is a translator, someone who can speak the words of healing and direction. Supa Nova Slom is that translator.

I believe *The Remedy* is an important foundational step in the path of wellness for our youth. I read the book from introduction to ending and believe it, in my medical opinion, to be foundationally sound and nutritionally worthy. The principles of wellness expounded by Supa Nova Slom are irrefutably the front-line "weapons of mass destruction" for the state of dis-ease. Of particular interest is how simply it is arranged, with consideration for the never-ending dilemma of how to eat healthy with limited funds.

I found it to be not only well-written, but spoken in a tone and manner that can be easily digested not only by Generations X, Y, and Z, but by Boomers, if they so choose.

I endorse it enthusiastically, with my professional imprimatur, and look forward to its implementation within my own practice in Brooklyn.

Bernadette L. Sheridan, MD, FAAFP
Brooklyn, New York
December 1, 2008

Foreword by Queen Afua

Supa Nova Slom, the hip-hop Medicine Man and originator of the Chlorophyllian lifestyle, has stepped forward to present *The Remedy* as a healing solution to our toxic and epidemic conditions. The Remedy promises to recharge, rejuvenate, restore, and harmonize the reader into body, mind, and spirit unity. Over the years I have watched in pure amazement as my firstborn son has embarked on a powerful journey as a second-generation community activist and wellness coach devoted to bringing wellness to the masses at home and abroad. His method of communicating has empowered me, and together we have become, as he calls it, Wellness Warriors. The Remedy is the result of Supa Nova's journey.

Supa Nova Slom was born in 1977, seven years after I embarked on my own journey of holistic healing beginning at seventeen. I raised my son at a time when the vegetarian lifestyle was rejected within my community and even more so in my family. "She's crazy, she's endangering the children, she's not a responsible parent, she's depriving her children of a normal life"—I heard it all. I had to battle with my parents, my children's father, and other family members every day. They had no concern whatsoever about giving my kids junk food, French fries, and animal flesh, despite that it made them sick. Through it all I felt protected and directed by nature to keep growing my children holistically.

At school Supa Nova was ashamed about being raised differently. The other kids ridiculed him and made fun of his lifestyle. Over time he began to rebel, eating candy and junk food like an addict. Green juices, organic food, and herbal teas and remedies were no match for the seductive poisons of the eighties junk-food generation. It wasn't long before his behavior began to match his addictions. He fell from grace and began lying, stealing, and keeping the wrong company.

After his life was threatened while running wild in the streets, I sent him away to stay with family down south. During his two years away, Supa Nova and I repaired our relationship and developed a strong bond as son and mother and as comrades in healing. The distance brought us closer, and all that I had taught him, and all he'd learned on his own, began to come together. When Supa Nova returned to Brooklyn I noticed that he was always carrying a gallon of green liquid. I finally asked him what the gallon of greens was all about. Supa Nova simply replied, "I'm a Chlorophyllian." He explained that a Chlorophyllian consumes 70 percent green foods and liquids and 30 percent whole grains, nuts, seeds, and fruits. He credited this gallon of green liquid for breaking his addiction to sugar and returning his emotional balance. I was so amazed by his lifestyle that one year later I followed in my own son's footsteps and became a Chlorophyllian too. I recognize this as the remedy that magnified my life to a higher plane, and have never turned back.

The Remedy is an inspirational holistic diet book for the new age. It guides us to seek out nature's pharmacy for relief and offers us a source of nourishment for body, mind, and spirit by embracing the green fields of herbs, plants, trees, leaves, fruits, berries, and seaweed for wellness. The Remedy teaches us to welcome these chlorophyll-rich green foods into our lives for cell growth, repair, and energy.

The power to heal is in the people. We can all mend our wounded souls, resculpt our bodies, heal ourselves from the challenges of the world, and rebuild ourselves from affected bloodlines and toxic encounters. As a wellness warrior and author of *Heal Thyself for Health & Longevity; Sacred Woman: A Guide to Healing the Feminine Body, Mind, and*

Spirit; and *The City of Wellness: Restoring Youth Health Through The Seven Kitchens of Consciousness,* I can attest to the fact that The Remedy teaches that when you consume whole foods, you create wholeness in your life.

It is a solid reminder that our remedies have always been and will always be in nature.

Even President Barack Obama acknowledges that this nation needs wellness programs in order to save lives and restore the economy. We as a nation are eating ourselves to death and using toxic fast food to comfort us through our pain. The medical cost is astronomical and the spiritual loss is simply heartbreaking. Thankfully, The Remedy has arrived to challenge the country and awaken the American conscience. To heal thyself is to embrace a lifestyle of wellness. This is the message put forth by The Remedy.

Introduction

I'm Supa Nova Slom, a second-generation health activist and educator brought up in Crown Heights, Brooklyn. My mother, Queen Afua, saw to it that my sister, my brother, and I were raised on life-giving vegetable juices and natural ingredients, and refrained from eating the poison foods, preservatives, and additives that most of the other kids in our hood scarfed down like there was no tomorrow. I've performed periodic body cleanses and detoxing fasts my whole life. We were doing yoga decades before it was something joked about on *Sex and the City*. In my household, the positive power and nearly unlimited energy that exercise, a healthy diet, and periodic fasting create was not a new phase or fad, it was a tradition. I have the blessing of health to show for it. What Mom was and is about is holistic wellness. Simply defined, holistic health:

* Seeks to prevent disease before it starts
* Recognizes that the body, mind, and spirit are one and that a problem with any one aspect of that trio affects the other two
* Assumes that health is a matter of lifestyle and the choices you make about how you live

The tradition and practice of holistic wellness goes back centuries, and the ideas that Queen Afua taught me have been in play since before recorded history. If there's one word that describes the principal goal of holistic health, it's balance. The ancients had scores of words and symbols to describe the delicate equilibrium between body, mind, and spirit. Balance—not neutrality, not inertia, not paralysis—is a dynamic, energetic, and healthy give-and-take that favors and flatters and enables the magically, beautifully, fabulously perfect systems that keep you alive to harmoniously flow and do their jobs.

It took the Industrial Revolution to mess up that balance and introduce many toxins into our system, but the modern holistic health movement has risen up to face these challenges. Fortunately, doctors, scientists, practitioners, and therapists from every background and ethnicity have begun to undo the damage and address both old and new ways to restore the body's long-recognized need for balanced health and well-being. Nutritionists have found that a diet dominated by green vegetables—an ideal source of vitamins, minerals, and enzymes, fiber for cleansing, and water for oxygenating and flushing the system—can restore internal balance and prolong lives threatened by an increasingly toxic environment.

Health practitioners have detailed the healing properties of blue green algae, prairie grasses like wheatgrass, and other specific fruits and vegetables that are now called *superfoods*. Juicing advocate Dr. Norman Walker, fasting expert Paul Bragg, and raw foodist Ann Wigmore have taken the discussion even further, and many of their ideas have been incorporated into my mom's citadel of wellness and been part of our holistic living for half a century. Coming up in the eighties, I not only was a poster child for this essential wisdom, I saw firsthand what happens when a body that craves green foods and proper nutrition is fed garbage. African Americans have led this country in the arts, sports, and politics for more than a century. Unfortunately, over the last three decades, black Americans have set the standard for poor health statistics. Urban neighborhoods of the eighties were the proving ground for the new wave of processed foods and fast foods that are now making Americans sick and tired everywhere in the country. African Americans were the guinea pigs for the processed food industry and pharmaceutical corporations that have sold the whole country on a lifestyle that doesn't use diet to prevent disease or slow aging—even though we live in one of the only civilized nations on Earth without national health care.

What Mom taught me and fed me made my body and spirit strong. Defending that lifestyle legacy made me tough. In the eighties, my hood was a hard place to stay healthy. From day one, I had to fight my own battle for wellness. Going to school during the years that Run-DMC was rapping on the radio about KFC and Big Macs, the sprout sandwich Queen packed for my lunch guaranteed confrontation. Kids don't like different, and there were days when I had to literally fight my way out of the cafeteria.

Home had its challenges, too. As a teenager, I divided my time between my father's apartment in the Cypress Hill projects and my mom's Crown Heights citadel of wellness. One weekend my stepmother would feed me grilled sandwiches made from toxic government cheese and oleo margarine, and the next weekend I'd be drinking my mother's pure vegetable juices. At the same time I was absorbing the principles of preventative nutrition, martial arts, yoga, meditation, and other foundations of holistic wellness from my mother's network of practitioners, I came to know thug life with its gangs, guns, and the dollars that make it all happen. That's where another family tradition kicked in.

Mom didn't just look after her own, she reached out to anyone, anywhere who was sick and tired of feeling sick and tired from the ravages of body toxins, obesity, and other Toxitarian diet-related illnesses. Gangsta life is as high-stress as any corner-office corporate gig. So when members of my crew were struggling with their weight, trying to keep their strength up to live large and hard and party the way they wanted to, I was there with the skills and tools and principles to help them stay on point through diet. Hungover? Strung out? I got that. Overstressed from scheming, dealing, and watching your back 24/7? Here's what you do . . . I was there with the goods and the facts and the means to restore balance and make sure my crew was able to live and earn and fight another day. That's when they started calling me the Medicine Man. I had the hookup for health.

When I took my first steps into the music industry, that name followed. The secret truth I discovered as a recording artist is that a balanced lifestyle of holistic wellness is something that's practiced by many of hip-hop's biggest names. Russell Simmons, the RZA and the GZA from Wu-Tang, and many other old-school rappers are devout vegans. Chuck D and Professor Griff from Public Enemy, Doug E. Fresh, Common, Andre 3000, and Erykah Badu have all benefited from Queen Afua's wisdom or have worked with me to keep themselves green-clean and green-strong inside and out. I've toured and performed and consulted with the best and I know what I'm talking about. The same "ride or die" mentality I learned on the street is what keeps hip-hop's biggest names at the top of their game. The secret truth I'm here to share with you is that for the kings and queens of hip-hop, no matter what the lyrics say and the videos show, backstage the mantra is "get healthy or die tryin'."

Cipher—in the hip-hop world it's a word that carries weight. A cipher is your circle—your crew, your world, the community of collaborators around you. That means a lot. As you live, move and create, you share all kinds of company with all kinds of people and travel through all kinds of scenes, neighborhoods, and communities. Working alongside my mom as she took her message of holistic wellness all over the country and the world, I passed through dozens of ciphers. Whether it was a Fort Greene charter school, a Marin County yoga retreat, or a suburban Atlanta community center, Queen Afua's message came through loud and clear. Alongside Mom and then on my own, first in gang circles, then hip-hop circles, then through outreach education and speaking engagements, I've learned firsthand that the principles and practices of holistic wellness can restore balance and energy in anyone's life. Now that the world is catching up to Mom's message and what used to be considered fringe beliefs have moved into the mainstream, the truth is even clearer.

To break free of gang life and its unhealthy temptations, I finished high school in Greensboro, North Carolina, where my aunt lived. That's where The Remedy truly took root. While working out, going to school, meditating, writing music, and generally getting myself together, I began to reflect on the various approaches to diet that I'd encountered up to then. Between Brooklyn, the capital of the Rastafarian Ital health movement and home of the Park Slope Food Coop, and my travels around the country, I'd encountered thousands of vegetarians. But when you looked in the shopping cart of many of them, the emphasis they put on prepackaged foods, grains, and starches made what they ate not that far different from what's making kids from DeKalb Avenue to Denver overweight and unhealthy.

The majority of vegetarians, I realized, were Starchitarians. Maybe they're not eating meat, or maybe they cut out dairy, but the bulk of their diet is still processed starches just like any Toxitarian, with all the preservatives, chemicals, and GMO ingredients, and all the health risks and potential for obesity those things bring. What Toxitarians and Starchitarians and the majority of Americans ignore is the cleansing and nutritive power of greens. Carnivore or vegan, overweight or underweight, the secret to cleansing and detoxifying and reenergizing your life is the same: *Eat green.*

Look no farther than the sun in the sky—that's where the energy starts. That's where the power comes from. That's what we use to jet through our days and nights in good health and full strength. The simple miracle of photosynthesis is the source of a remedy that revs up human cells, cleanses and oxygenates human blood, and keeps us kicking and popping and taking our lives to the next level no matter how much stress we take on and no matter what age we are.

You picked up this book looking to get thin and get going? You can only get well if you stop poisoning yourself with toxic foods, start cleansing your body of the ravages we all face from the environment, and start giving yourself and your cells what you really need—a concentrated dose of the sun's radiant energy captured in the nutrient-dense cells of green plant foods.

Over the next seven chapters I'm going to lay out a program that begins with using the power of the sun and the miracle of photosynthesis to restore your natural heritage of unlimited energy, physical strength, mental sharpness, and sexual potency and end the self-inflicted illness and accompanying weight gain of a toxic diet.

My program has two stages:

Part 1—The Remedy

A four-day detox that revitalizes as it cleanses, and restores balance by flushing and feeding your body.

Part 2—The Five-Week Supa Power Plan

A structured meal and exercise plan designed to phase out toxic ingredients and additives in the food you eat, rid your body of accumulated food poisons, combat the fat, and put you in the groove and on point to a longer, healthier life.

Along with a schedule and recipes, both these stages will include the same idea ingredients:

THE TRUTH—Examines the history and facts behind the steps we'll take together.

WHAT'S GOOD?—Lists the foods, ingredients, and other tools you'll need in order to put the plan into action.

THE WORD—Features testimony and advice from some of the biggest and most influential names behind the scenes and on stage in hip-hop.

THE BODY—Puts the renewed energy to use in a series of exercises designed to assist your body in cleansing itself through moving, breathing, and sweating, and strengthen you as you go.

THE LOVE—Incorporates six motivational principles I've found to be inseparable from healing, cleansing, and getting in shape holistically:

1. Will and Desire
2. Self-Love and Appreciation

3. Activation
4. Discipline
5. Emotional healing
6. Faith

The Love affirms the facts of The Truth, the value of What's Good?, the wisdom of The Word, and the unlimited resiliency of The Body. The Love brings it all together—it syncopates all the rhythms and moves you make. In a word: *balance!* The Love is about taking the new positive energy and attitude of The Remedy to your family and out to your community and the world. It may seem like diet and exercise are all about you, but The Love says otherwise. By the time we're done, you'll know how it feels to be clean, green, lean, and open to the opportunities and pleasures and blessings of a balanced, healthy life lived to its fullest.

PART I

The Remedy

one

The Remedy Chlorophyllian Cleanse

"The eyes are the window to the soul."

True talk. When you look into someone's eyes you catch a glimpse of the world of feelings and ideas percolating inside them. But those eyes are also a window on health. Have a look at the whites of your eyes in a mirror. Not very white, are they? A touch yellowed? Plenty of visible blood vessels? Have that too-shiny and glazed look, a dry yet slick feeling when you blink and a kind of dull ache when you pinch them shut?

Your eyes reveal what's physically going on inside you. The yellowing, the foggy glaze, the tired, squeaky blinking, the general cotton-lidded sensation you get as you prop your eyes open and hold your body upright at work and at play are signs that your liver, kidneys, immune system, and other internal organs and processes are working beyond peak capacity to filter out impurities and make something useful out of the Toxitarian diet you eat.

It's the same with your skin. Your body's single largest organ offers a similar look inside. Gently pinch the skin on your cheek, near your eye. Does it feel smooth and soft between your fingers? Does it slip right back into place with a gentle elasticity? No? It can. But the skin can't adequately renew itself, can't breathe, maintain softness, age, and heal gradually, if it's covering up a disaster area of overtaxed organs, dehydrated cells, and tired, oxygen-starved blood.

❑ Lack of energy
❑ Obesity
❑ Glassy, foggy eyes
❑ Prematurely wrinkled, oily or dry skin, and/or acne
❑ Brittle hair
❑ Yellow nails
❑ Bad breath and body odor
❑ Irritability and mood swings
❑ Inability to concentrate
❑ Food cravings
❑ Mucous membrane irritation and extreme allergy symptoms

All of these issues stem from the same source—body toxicity. All of them can be treated, improved, and even alleviated by the same technique—cleansing and detoxifying the body and getting your cells the pure, natural nutrient fuel they need. The goal of The Remedy Four-Day Chlorophyllian Cleanse is to give you a simple, easy, surefire way to detoxify, clean, and recharge your body's internal organs and start the journey to a more energized, sleeker, healthier you.

THE TRUTH

Human beings, like all animals, are consumers and transformers. I'm not talking about comparison shopping for flat-screen TVs or turning from a car into a robot and back again. We're made of billions of individual cells that consume food and transform it into energy 24/7, from the moment we're conceived until we die, and even after we die, in the case of the cells that make up our hair and fingernails.

Cells are specialists. Every one of the trillions of cells that we're composed of has a specific function it is programmed to perform. And each tiny little cell in us, regardless of its specialty, is looking to get fed in order to ramp up, grow, and make more of itself and do the job it was created to do. Any human cell, skin cell, pancreas cell, hair cell, brain cell, or whatever cell is looking to eat well. What a cell needs is to live and grow and function in a balanced environment that's naturally rich in the vitamins, minerals, amino acids, enzymes, and other nutrients and natural chemicals it craves. The cell's ideal cipher is a place where the right amino acids, glucose for energy, oxygen, and other natural substances will float by so that the enzymes within the cell can snatch them inside through the permeable cell wall and put them to use as energy and to make other tools to perform that cell's specialty function.

Convenience, mass production, rapid travel, and all the other benefits we take for granted in the modern age have come at a steep price. Burning fossil fuels trashes the air we all breathe. Manufacturing, especially plastics, and operating massive factory farms to produce livestock, dairy, and inorganically grown vegetable ingredients for processed foods and for our tables dumps literally tons of deadly toxins in the water we all need to survive and grow. Most of us take that constant assault even further by ingesting the additives, hormones, dyes, and preservatives (along with excess calories) in processed foods, fast food, and heavy meat and dairy Toxitarian diets. Add to that the toxic chemical compounds in the cosmetic soaps, moisturizers, and beauty products women and, increasingly, men slather onto their porous, breathing skins and you have a body under siege from toxicity at all times and from all directions.

The human body has an amazing capacity for storing, combining, and utilizing nutrients, flushing out excess and cleansing itself of impurities and potentially toxic substances it may absorb along with the good stuff. We flush out the bad when we:

* Exhale
* Sweat
* Urinate/defecate
* Slough off dead skin

The natural process of excretion, via deep breathing, breaking a sweat, and going to the bathroom can always use help. Nearly every culture on earth has adopted some kind of cleansing and detoxing technique. Our forebears made rituals out of emptying the lungs, sweating out toxins, and rinsing out the colon and lower intestine.

* Fasting for religious reasons
* Ritual sweating, from *shvitz* (orthodox Jews) to sweat lodge (Native Americans)
* Exercise
* Colon cleansing via colonics or enemas

All these things have a very welcome detoxifying effect on the body and help to maintain a high level of energy and a healthy body weight.

Today we're more inclined to make a ritual out of taking in toxicity! Every trip to the drive-thru, every cigarette, every gulp of a soda or a beer smuggles harmful ingredients into our bodies and cultivates illness, obesity, and exhaustion. Our bodies need help ridding us of the things we ritually and voluntarily put inside it.

There are three basic issues at work here:

1. Your body needs to be detoxed.
   The voluntary intake of toxins through food has to stop.
2. Your body needs to be cleansed.
   The body's natural flushing processes need a major boost.
3. Your body needs a Supa Dose of nutrition.
   You must feed your consuming and transforming cells what they must have in order to live.

Before we go into a five-week power plan designed to control and curtail the voluntary consumption of the things that make us sick, tired, and overweight, and boost the body's own filtering and flushing ways, let's kick-start the detox.

THE WORD

Hype Williams is one of hip-hop's true innovators. First as a tagger and graffiti artist, then as a graphic designer and finally an award-winning, groundbreaking, and prolific video, commercial, and film director, Brother Hype has defined a look and the motion of hip-hop and R&B that has influenced a generation.

"It's just a struggle across the board," Hype says about his desire to stay healthy. "Especially when you realize the kind of advertising that's out there. People are bombarded with food twenty-four hours a day—TV, billboards, there's like twenty restaurants on every block. You struggle with it. Half the time my mentality is clear, but just like anybody else, I get bombarded with all of this food and bad lifestyle and bad living in the company you keep and the media.

"Some people smoke cigarettes," Hype says, "some people smoke weed, or drink or eat pork and beef and refined sugar and all that stuff. I try to fight that by completely abstaining from food three times a year. Once you attempt to get it out of your system, you see that there's a difference in how your body operates without that stuff in it. If you don't do some kind of seasonal fast for religious purposes, there are alternatives. You just gotta give it a shot to see the difference in how you feel. It's like anything else. When you get some really good sleep, like that good sleep when you wake up, like that feeling versus an average night's sleep, it's a different thing."

THE TRUTH

All human cells want food containing the amino acids, water, vitamins, and minerals they're craving, but that our bodies can't produce on our own—enzymes that will assist the cells' own consuming and transforming, and provide oxygen to help keep things popping. But our cells and the organ systems they make up also need to have all that good stuff on hand in a body environment with a pH balance that's sympathetic to the whole transformation process.

Strictly defined, pH is the ratio of acid (the positively charged, atomically grabby half of the two-part molecular dance that makes up chemical compounds) to alkali (the "base," or negatively charged, more stable, and atomically generous half of the same team) inside us. When acid and alkali are in balance in the human body, everything is on a harmonious smooth cruise to a long healthy life—what since the 1920s has become known as *homeostasis*. But when we start to rip off our cells' expectations by feeding them Toxitarian garbage like meat, dairy, sugar, simple starches, excess sodium, alcohol, and the rogues' gallery of artificial and unnatural preservatives and chemicals in processed foods, we invariably tip things over to the acid side.

Acid pH foods include:

* Processed grains and simple starches like bleached white flour and white-flour baked goods
* Deep-fried anything
* Animal protein like beef, pork, chicken, turkey, fish, and eggs
* Hydrogenated oils, animal fats, and butter
* Dairy foods like milk, cheese, and ice cream
* All refined and added sugars
* Alcohol like beer, wine, and spirits and drugs like tobacco and marijuana
* Aspirin, and most over-the-counter and prescription oral medications
* Chemical additives like salt and other preservatives
* Pesticides absorbed from nonorganic produce and from meat raised on sprayed crops

The first ingredient necessary to restore the body's proper pH balance and homeostasis is water—a lot of it. You cannot thrive or even survive without the water your body needs. Every schoolkid knows that the human body itself is upwards of 70 percent water. That percentage needs to be maintained at all times, which requires A LOT of water. The water in your body is constantly working—in motion, moving from cell to cell, organ to organ, flushing, oxygenating, and keeping you clean. The life-giving oxygen in water is an essential part of every single one of your body's metabolic and cellular processes. Of course, we breathe in oxygen all day and night. It arrives in our lungs in a cocktail composed mostly of nitrogen, carbon dioxide, and, for the last couple centuries anyway, increasing amounts of nasty Industrial Age pollution that we put into our air when we burn and make things. But O_2-hungry cells also get oxygen from the food we eat and water we drink. Water is the wonder drug, the magic bullet. When you constantly hydrate your body with pure, clean water, your system gets a flush boost, giving it the best possible advantage against toxins and a bad diet.

It's dramatic what happens when you actually meet the body's water requirement. Even if you choose only to supplement a poor diet with double the intake of water you drink now, you'd see a difference in your eyes, skin, and hair after just a few days. When your body is getting all the water it needs (probably about twice what you're giving it now), even if the rest of what you put into you is fast-food garbage, your skin and eyes will improve in clarity, your digestion will run more smoothly, and you'll feel stronger and better in every department.

THE WORD

"You must drink and maintain a certain intake of water," says Tyson Beckford. "It naturally flushes the body and keeps you right." My Brother knows of what he speaks. His body and face are his livelihood. Since he broke out in the modeling scene of the early nineties, Tyson's athletic frame and exotic looks have helped him to refocus and redefine the masculine media image. Whether as the face of Ralph Lauren, one of *People's* exalted 50 Most Beautiful People, the key visual ingredient in dozens of music videos, print ads, and films, or as cohost of *Make Me a Super-model*, Tyson Beckford commands attention and respect because he pays attention and respect to his body.

"A good glass of water puts you in a better mood," Tyson says. "People don't realize that a lot of stuff they put into themselves every day is not right, you know? The sugar and the artificial flavoring and color, that stuff takes a toll on your body. Look at your insides as if they were a white linen shirt. You put anything other than water on white linen, pour any coloring on it and it's going to stain, right? Your intestines and your stomach lining, your whole digestive tract is colored by those different artificial flavors and man-made coloring that the body's not used to and not designed to take." Brother Tyson's challenge? "Put yourself on a water diet for thirty days," he says. "Go thirty days drinking just water with breakfast instead of having juice or coffee. Drink water every time you're thirsty, eight glasses a day, and don't drink any soda. You'll notice how your body will change and how much better you'll feel in those thirty days."

WHAT'S GOOD?

"Water," according to Brother Tyson Beckford, "is the simplest and easiest thing to buy. It doesn't have to cost you a whole lot of money to buy yourself a gallon of water, walk around with that, and knock that out." Unfortunately, the quickest and easiest way to get water is also one of the most suspect. Tap water contains the additive fluoride. Fluoride is a toxic metal and to be avoided (as much as this country's crazy fluoridation policy will let you). Also, most American water treatment plants are not equipped to filter out the pesticide run-off from toxic factory farm agriculture, which makes tap water even more dubious. Does that mean your water needs to be from Fiji? No, it just needs to be clean. Boutique bottled waters can cost a lot of money. Tap water is out. What does that leave?

* Alkaline water—supplemented with negative ions so that it is high-alkaline. It's great for you, but it can be expensive.
* Commercially bottled spring and artesian well waters—some are cheap, some aren't. Bottled water is still a boutique item, compared to tap water, and can sometimes have purity issues.
* Home-filtered water—Brita, PÛR, etc. It's cheap, after the initial investment in the pitcher and the regular replacement of the filter. But the filter on a Brita can only keep out so much. It does nothing to remove fluoride, for instance.
* Distilled water—converted to steam, removing impurities and minerals in the process. Distilled water has my vote for best all-around value and purity for the buck.

THE TRUTH

Breathing and oxygen-rich water consumed on its own and used in our food play a huge part in helping us rid our body of toxins. But in order to flush, detox, and revive with the Remedy Four-Day Cleanse, you'll need the biggest nutritional oxygen boost of all—chlorophyll.

Plants thrive on nutrients from the soil they live in, oxygen from the air and water they take in, and light from the sun. The miraculous process by which those things harmoniously foster healthy cell growth in plants is called, as we all learned in grade school, photosynthesis. Chlorophyll, a combination of molecules making up the green parts of the plant, is what makes photosynthesis possible. Human beings ingest plant chlorophyll, and the accompanying enzymes and nutrients that make plants grow, when we eat any leafy green vegetables.

In the human body, chlorophyll-rich foods restore pH and promote the vital disbursement of oxygen in the bloodstream. Chlorophyll, the "blood" of the plant, acts like a transfusion of nutrients, amino acids, and enzymes that we need to keep our blood healthy and pumped full of oxygen. Studies increasingly indicate that chlorophyll-rich plant foods help cells to restore damage to their DNA codes and replicate healthily. A pH-balanced stomach full of chlorophyll digests better, passes waste more efficiently, and cuts your liver and other hardworking vital organs miles of slack. Many of the physical symptoms and ravages of a lifestyle that embraces bad food can be treated and improved by a diet rich in chlorophyll.

All green vegetables contain chlorophyll. The greener they are, the more chlorophyll-rich they are. But since meat and dairy, food additives, polluted air, and other environmental body hazards put us in the toxic crosshairs at all times, we need to flush and combat those poisons with an extra-potent dose of the green stuff. That's where blue-green algae comes into the fight. Marketed and consumed as spirulina, chlorella "green food," "green juice," or "pure liquid chlorophyll" supplements, this commercially available chlorophyll-rich superfood acts like body armor, slowing down and stopping those toxin bullets that would otherwise rip through your immune system, digestion, heart, liver, lungs, brain, and muscles.

Taken as a supplement (powder, liquid, or tablet), spirulina and chlorella supercharge your blood and immune system to a degree unrivaled by just about any other food source. Regular consumption of any combination of these algae food supplements also helps the body's ongoing efforts to purge itself of toxic environmental contaminants and balance pH to sustain homeostasis. Blue-green algae also stimulates the growth of the T cells and white blood cells that the immune system uses to fight illness. It also evens out blood pressure and blood sugar. When it's grown and harvested in a pure, clean, and consistently nutrient-balanced state beneficial to human consumption, blue-green algae contains vegetarian amino acid protein to feed your hungry cells; essential fatty acids for the heart; enzymes, beneficial bacteria, and fiber to give your stomach, bowels, and liver a hand up; and antioxidant vitamins (like naturally occurring B12) galore.

The other all-powerful chlorophyll-powered supplements are prairie grasses, such as wheatgrass, alfalfa, and barley grass. In the first half of the twentieth century, nutritionists began extolling the virtues of wheatgrass and the incredibly dense cocktail of chlorophyll, enzymes, and minerals within it. By pressing the juice out of the immature grassy shoots of the wheat berry plant, and other grasses that grow naturally on the American prairie, wheatgrass advocates created a very strong, very green, very powerful nutritional supplement. Whether via a fresh shot at a juice bar, or taken in concentrated powdered form, wheatgrass and the other prairie grasses like alfalfa and green barley grass are an incredibly intense and healthy solar energy booster. Wheat berry, alfalfa, and green barley grass juices are loaded with calcium, amino acid protein, and an abundance of vitamins, minerals, and enzymes that strengthen the skeleton, build muscle, boost the immune system, and help the body cleanse itself. All told, wheatgrass juice contains every vitamin, mineral, and enzyme needed to sustain human life.

When I was putting myself back together in North Carolina, I was also putting The Remedy together. Mom had turned me on to consuming chlorophyll from spirulina, chlorella, and prairie grass juices in concentrated supplement form as a kid. As I grew older, I found the energy boost so invigorating and powerful that I would take a gallon jug of distilled water, pop the cap, spoon in a mixture of powered greens that I had made, shake it up, and then drink down the gallon over the course of a day. Studying, working out—everywhere I went, the jug went with me. When I returned to Brooklyn, the jug and my daylong green juice ritual came along, too. Between the jug and a diet composed almost completely of deep-colored, chlorophyll-rich vegetables and fruits, I had moved beyond vegetarian or vegan—I had become a Chlorophyllian!

WHAT'S GOOD?

Eventually I decided that I should tailor my own mixture of chlorophyll supplements. I experimented with various combinations of powdered greens, and eventually came up with the Supa Mega Greens formula. My particular Chlorophyllian supplement body, soul, and cell feast incorporates seven different green foods and herb ingredients:

✓ Spirulina

✓ Sun chlorella

✓ Sea greens rich in chlorophyll, phytochemicals (more on those later), vitamins, minerals, protein, and enzymes

✓ Wheatgrass

✓ Alfalfa grass

✓ Green barley grass

✓ Concentrated prairie grasses. These powdered grasses pack a nutrient-dense and cleansing wallop. They supercharge your cells, boost your immune system, and oxygenate the blood. They also deodorize your insides and improve the smell of your breath and sweat while removing toxins and restoring your body's ideal pH.

Plus:

✓ Ginger

✓ Dandelion

Ginger root adds flavor, has antibacterial properties, revs up bile production in the gallbladder, soothes the stomach, and helps to cleanse the blood. In concentrated powder form, dandelion greens help to drain toxins that weigh down immune function while also restoring and preserving pH.

THE TRUTH

My whole life I've done juice fasts, the Master Cleanse, water fasts—almost every kind of fast and cleanse that there is—and I can personally attest to the fact The Remedy cleanse program is the greatest, quickest, and easiest mental, physical, emotional, and spiritual natural reboot I've found to date.

CLEANSE BENEFITS	MASTER CLEANSE	AÇAI BERRY CLEANSE	JUICE FAST	WATER FAST	THE REMEDY
Detoxifies	Yes	Yes	Yes	Yes	**Yes**
Cleanses	Yes	Yes	Yes	Yes	**Yes**
Nutrient dense	No	Yes	Yes	No	**Yes**
Quick and easy	No	No	No	No	**Yes**
Simple	No	Yes	No	Yes	**Yes**
Potential side effects	Many	Many	Few	Many	**Few**

Over the course of The Remedy Four-Day Chlorophyllian Cleanse, you will:

* Detox
* Flush
* Cleanse
* Oxygenate
* Feed
* Energize

The Remedy's gentle but thorough program:

✓ Increases energy
✓ Sharpens mental clarity
✓ Gives relief to mucous membrane symptoms
✓ Clears up skin and eyes, and restores luster to hair and nails
✓ Eases up on your digestive tract and gets your bowels flowing
✓ Encourages your body to rid itself of excess weight

I know that last point is a big one for a lot of you. Depending on your weight and your level of toxicity at the start, strictly following The Remedy Four-Day Chlorophyllian Cleanse will help you to lose weight.

Weight Loss Goals:

* Toxitarian: 4–11 pounds
* Starchitarian: 4–8 pounds
* Strict Vegetarian/Vegan/Chlorophyllian: 3–6 pounds

NOTE: These numbers are GOALS. Your actual results will depend on:

* Metabolism
* The specifics of your diet going into the cleanse
* Your weight, height, age, and body mass index (BMI) at the time of the cleanse
* How active you are before and during the cleanse

There are no hard, fast rules about weight loss with The Remedy, just as there are no hard, fast rules about weight loss with any cleanse.

NOTE: As with any cleanse, regardless of your health goals or physical condition, you should consult with your doctor before undertaking The Remedy Four-Day Chlorophyllian Cleanse.

WHAT'S GOOD?

The Remedy Four-Day Cleanse has just three basic ingredients:

1. Two 12-ounce glasses of fruit juice a day for four days + one recovery day
2. One gallon jug of distilled water per day for four days + one recovery day
3. Five heaping tablespoons of Supa Mega Greens per day for four days + one recovery day

Looking at it as a grocery list, you'll simply need to buy:

* Two 64-ounce containers of juice
* Four gallon jugs of water
* Ingredients for Supa Mega Greens

Supa Mega Greens

1 tsp. spirulina
1 tsp. sun chlorella
1 tsp. powdered wheatgrass (or 3 oz. of fresh wheatgrass juice)
1 tsp. powdered alfalfa grass (or 3 oz. fresh alfalfa grass juice)
1 tsp. powdered green barley grass (or 3 oz. fresh green barley grass juice)
½ tsp. fresh ginger, juiced (two or three decent-sized fingers of fresh
    ginger should do it)
1 cup dandelion greens, juiced or powdered

Mix ingredients in a separate container, then add to gallon jug of water.

My Supa Mega Greens powder combines low-temperature dehydrated, highly concentrated forms of these fresh juices and greens and is available from www.supanovaslom.com.

Juice

Ideally, you should use fresh-squeezed juice from organic sources. Cold pressing—the slow crushing of juice from fruit—is the best process, because it gets the maximum yield and doesn't mix excess air into the juice the way that other mechanical juicers do. The reality of course is that almost no one has a cold-press juicer in their home, and even those with cheaper electric juicers on hand can find it difficult to work juicing into their schedule. Your real-world juice source options are as follows:

✓ Best: Fresh-squeezed or cold-pressed from organically grown fruit
✓ Okay: Fresh-squeezed from nonorganic fruit

✓ Passable: Bottled or carton juice that has not been reconstituted or made from concentrate

✓ If you must: Reconstituted or from-concentrate juice

Not acceptable:

✗ ANY juice product with ANY sugar additives (fructose, corn syrup, added white grape juice; any ingredient other than the juice from the fruit that's pictured and named on the carton). That includes all "juice drinks" and most juice blends. The Remedy won't work if you toxify with sugar and other added ingredients.

For a first-time Remedy Cleanse experience, I find that it helps to pick a variety of juices according to these categories:

DAY 1. ENTICE JUICES—FLAVORS YOU PARTICULARLY LIKE

✓ Orange
✓ Pineapple
✓ Grapefruit
✓ Tangerine

DAY 2. SUBACID JUICES—JUICES FROM FRUIT WITH A HIGH-ALKALI PH

✓ Apple (not sour apple)
✓ Pear
✓ Grape
✓ Cherry
✓ Cranberry (the juice, not the sweetened drink kind)
✓ Blackberry
✓ Prune

✓ Apricot
✓ Peach
✓ Kiwi
✓ Pomegranate
✓ Açai berry

DAY 3. MELON JUICE–SWEET AND SOOTHING

✓ Cantaloupe
✓ Honeydew
✓ Watermelon

If you can't find fresh melon juices in the supermarket, try a farmers' market or organic grocery, or juice your own with a juicer.

DAY 4. TROPICAL FRUIT

✓ Papaya
✓ Mango
✓ Guava

Water

Like I said, I prefer distilled water to boutique bottled water. I find the gallon jug with the handle (the ones that look just like a gallon milk container) really convenient. The jug also has a nice heft and size that helps to remind you of your goals and the task at hand. When hard-core bodybuilders do intense training in the gym, they're never without a gallon plastic jug. On The Remedy, you're doing intense cell building, so let the world know you're hard-core by carrying the jug.

The downside of the gallon plastic jug of water is that the specific plastic used to manufacture those bottles is potentially hazardous and toxic on its own. Nalgene plastic bottles contain a chemical called bisphenol A (or BPA) which remains in the body and is thought to contribute to a variety of potentially fatal disorders. Health advocates say that the amount of BPA that leaches out of plastic water bottles is a cause for concern.

The Park Slope Food Coop in my native Brooklyn considers the risk serious enough that they no longer carry water bottled in plastic. The chemical industry—and for the most part, the government—say of course there's little or no risk to humans from the amount of BPA we absorb from a plastic jug. I'm on the fence. Part of The Remedy philosophy is that you can always do better; that your health and your well-being can always be improved. My feeling is that the additional cleansing and detoxing benefits of The Remedy cancel out the BPA risk, but you may feel differently. If so, you'll need to find an alternative gallon jug or you'll have to mix up the Supa Mega Green mix and gallon of water separately and put them in individual non-plastic bottles. Your move.

THE PLAN

Each day of The Remedy is divided into:

* A 6–9 A.M. breakfast period
* A 9 A.M.–5 P.M. all-day lunch period
* A 5–7 P.M. dinner period.

You may need to adapt the times to fit your waking hours, but the general breakdown of your uptime remains the same:

* Fruit juice and Supa Mega Greens at the start of your day.
* A gallon of water with Supa Mega Greens consumed for the middle eight hours of your day.

* Another fruit juice and Supa Mega Greens liquid meal when you would ordinarily have your last meal of the day.

DAY 1

Supa Liquid Breakfast Meal: 6–9 A.M.
12 ounces of freshly pressed organic fruit juice or unsweetened bottled juice with 1 heaping tablespoon of Supa Mega Greens

Supa All-Day Liquid Meal: 9 A.M.–5 P.M.
Tonic Mix: Add two heaping tablespoons of Supa Mega Greens to 1 gallon of distilled, filtered, or alkaline water.

Supa Liquid Dinner Meal: 5–7 P.M.
12 ounces of freshly pressed organic fruit juice or unsweetened bottled juice with 1–2 heaping tablespoons of Supa Mega Greens

DAY 2

Supa Liquid Breakfast Meal: 6–9 A.M.

Supa All-Day Liquid Meal: 9 A.M.–5 P.M.

Supa Liquid Dinner Meal: 5–7 P.M.

DAY 3

Supa Liquid Breakfast Meal: 6–9 A.M.

Supa All-Day Liquid Meal: 9 A.M.–5 P.M.

Supa Liquid Dinner Meal: 5–7 P.M.

DAY 4

Supa Liquid Breakfast Meal: 6–9 A.M.

Supa All-Day Liquid Meal: 9 A.M.–5 P.M.

Supa Liquid Dinner Meal: 5–7 P.M.

DAY 5—ENDING THE CLEANSE

First Remedy End Cleanse Meal

Supa Liquid Breakfast Meal: 6–9 A.M.

Along with breakfast: 6–8 ounces of fresh fruit—NOT canned or sweetened

Second Remedy End Cleanse Meal

Supa All-Day Liquid Meal: 9 A.M.–5 P.M.

Augment the gallon of water with a lunch of 6 ounces of warm (not hot) clear broth soup, such as miso.

Third and Final Remedy End Cleanse Meal

Supa Liquid Dinner Meal: 5–7 P.M.

Add a dinner of 1 cup of raw salad greens (Boston, iceberg, arugula, spinach, etc.) with the juice of ½ lemon used as dressing. NO tomatoes, onions, bottled dressing, or anything else.

The following day you may return to eating normally.

THE TRUTH

Like other cleanses, The Remedy greatly restricts your caloric intake along with your intake of potentially harmful food substances. Also, like other cleanses, it flushes out accumulated toxic elements your body has stored in its tissues. But unlike many other cleanses, The Remedy is putting back as it's taking out. The Supa Mega Greens mixture is oxygenating and bathing your cells in Chlorophyllian nutrition. The green juice powder is truly a tonic for organs and systems thrown out of whack by prior Toxitarian diet extremes.

And, since The Remedy is only a four-day program, it's much easier to stick to and has almost no side effects, such as the constipation, skin breakouts, irritability, and other problems associated with longer fasts.

THE BODY

The Remedy Cleanse flushes toxins from your body when you go to the bathroom, sweat, and breathe. To take full advantage of this likely overdue cleaning-out, pamper your skin and wash with extra care. Hot soaks and baths will help your skin rejuvenate.

Day 1: Dissove 1–4 tablespoons of Epsom salts or 1–2 tablespoons of sea salt into a hot bath and gently massage your entire body with a loofah or seaweed sponge and some oatmeal scrub from the health food store. Lightly scrubbing off the dead skin will increase your circulation and allow your skin to make the most of the cleanse.

Day 2: Moisten a sponge or loofah, apply oatmeal scrub, and wash your entire body in a warm shower.

Day 3: Soak your feet in a tub of water with 1 tablespoon Epsom salts in it. Remove one foot at a time and massage it with a pumice stone. After you're done, rub down feet, toes, and ankles with olive or castor oil.

Day 4: Epsom salt bath once again.

Supa Breath Work-In

Each day during the cleanse take a few moments to practice conscious breathing.

* Sit cross-legged on a mat or clean wood floor. Place your hands so that they rest gently on your knees.
* Relax your legs—just let them be where they feel least active and most comfortable within the crossed pose.
* Lengthen your spine—starting from the area just below your navel, gently draw your torso back and up until you feel at an unforced full height. It should be as if a string is hung down vertically through from the top of your head to your tailbone.
* Allow your shoulders to relax and drop naturally.

* Gently roll your neck to either side until it is relaxed.
* Bring your chin up.
* Quiet your mind—reach out mentally only as far as the energy and presence you feel in the moment, not the past, or what you may have to deal with later.
* Now, slowly inhale through your nose, letting your lungs fill from the bottom up as if you were pouring air into you like water from a pitcher. Once your lungs are full, pause for a moment and then purposefully exhale through your mouth at the same slow rate, emptying the top, middle, and finally the bottom of your lungs.

Repeat ten times for Day One, twenty for Day Two, thirty for Day Three, and forty for Day Four.

"I just can't do it!"

If you've successfully done a longer, more drastic cleanse, you'll find The Remedy a lot easier to complete. On The Remedy, the extra energy that sometimes doesn't kick in for days with other cleanses is there from the start. The Supa Mega Greens are so nutritionally pleasing to your body that it requires less active concentration to stick with the program for the full four days. Food cravings are minimal—the middle-of-the-day gallon-jug infusion will fill you up, no doubt.

Nevertheless, some people struggle with The Remedy. If you hit the wall the first day, try replacing the gallon of distilled water/Supa Mega Greens with an equal quantity of unsweetened coconut water with Supa Mega Greens dissolved in it. Find a store that sells unsweetened coconut water (no pulp) in the larger cartons rather than those little sippy-sized ones, so you don't have extra trash to recycle. The Remedy can be done one, two, three, or all four days with coconut water instead of distilled water. The effects may not be quite as dramatic as with the plain H_2O but you're still very likely to feel and look substantially better after following through to day five and after.

Another thing you can do the first day or two is flavor the all-day liquid meal jug with stevia. Though it's used on nearly half the sweetened processed foods in Japan (a country that banned aspartame, the active ingredient in NutraSweet), Israel (one of the most health-conscious countries on Earth), and much of the rest of the world, stevia—a natural sweetening extract made from a South American bush in the Chrysanthemum family, is almost unknown in the United States. Stevia is commercially available as both a spoonable granular powder and as a liquid. You can find it in most health food stores (the FDA only approves its sale as a food *supplement*, not a food *additive* like aspartame, so look for it next to the vitamins) and it can be purchased online. A few drops of the liquid version will sweeten your jug considerably.

And if you suffer from extremely high blood pressure, hypoglycemia, Type I or Type II diabetes, or are under an MD's or psychiatrist's care for an ongoing illness or condition, you should NOT undertake the cleanse without getting your doctor's permission. For the majority of people, The Remedy runs smoothly and safely, but if you experience:

* Extensive stomach cramps or bowel discomfort
* Diarrhea or constipation
* Headaches
* Nausea
* Dizziness
* Body aches or chills

or have been prone to those things in the past, stop the cleanse immediately and consult your doctor.

Okay, go back to the mirror and look at the whites of your eyes again. Notice an improvement? With less toxicity to contend with and a Supa Dose of chlorophyll nutrition to feed on, your liver, blood, immune system, brain, and other organs and processes have had a chance to regroup. Over the course of those four days, your body probably drew closer to its natural and correct pH than it's been since you were breast-fed. The cool, clear white cast your eyes have taken over the four-day cleanse and one-day recovery are a sign that walking the Chlorophyllian walk agrees with you.

Take a gentle pinch of your skin again. Feels different, right? Smoother, softer, more resilient? The signs are on you everywhere. Waistband a little looser? Bowels a little more regular? Less mucous discharge if you suffer from allergies? Less tension and fog on the brain? The Remedy Four-Day Chlorophyllian Cleanse is like that.

THE LOVE

The way I look at it, everything is food. Every word we hear, every touch we experience, every relationship affects us the same way food does: What the conscious mind ingests during the day, the unconscious digests while we sleep at night. The memory stores experiences, both toxic and nourishing, in the brain and feeds off of, or tries to flush, their good and bad ingredients as we go through our lives. Ideas? Food for thought. Music? *Food for the soul.* When we make love, when we exercise, when we relax and listen to the world inside us and out, we are consuming experience and transforming it into sensation and memory the same way that our cells consume nutrients and use them to transform.

When you eat and live toxically, it's because you're eating and living unconsciously. Consciously preparing a salad or doing a cleanse, or unconsciously sleepwalking to a burger joint or polishing off a quart bottle of soda, you run your life through choices. Doing anything, whether it's making the same mistake for the 1,000th time or a first step toward improvement, requires you to choose. All choices, good or bad, are governed by the same straightforward series of guiding principles and assumptions. In order to live consciously, make the right eating choices, and live your life well, healthy, and happy, you have to know what those guiding principles are, and use them to do the right thing.

There is no such thing as an absence of will and desire.

You are either exerting a will and desire to neglect yourself, to remain helpless and unconscious, or you are exerting a will and desire to get better, do well, and grow powerful and strong. The logical first step to free your mind is to commit to surviving and maximizing what years you have left on the planet.

One of the greatest benefits of The Remedy Cleanse is that it gives you a chance to reconnect with your body's healthy, balanced rhythms. As you prepare your juice and jug, drink The Remedy, flush toxins and fat, and clean yourself, listen to your body. Throughout The Remedy Cleanse and for the duration of the Supa Power Plan, keep a notebook and write down the thoughts and impressions you have. How do you feel physically and emotionally as you go about your day during the cleanse? What feels different? What's the same? How do your eyes look? Does the texture of your hair improve week to week? Are your dreams at night particularly vivid? Have your bathroom habits altered? Listen to your body and make note of what it is saying. In order to do that, you have one more fasting goal:

For the four nights of The Remedy Cleanse, don't watch TV. With that source of noise out of the picture, you'll be able to pick up on what your body is saying that much more easily.

The holistic lifestyle community relies a lot on affirmations. Café Gratitude, a dope chain of Bay Area vegan restaurants, uses a positive phrase to name every item on their menu. Their live-food veggie burger is called "I Am Cheerful." To order a lemonade with that, you say to your server, "I Am Refreshed," just like it says on the menu. What the owner of Café Gratitude and other holistic health advocates know is the same thing that psychologists, religious leaders, coaches, and motivational speakers have all discovered over the centuries—finding the words to describe a goal and saying them out loud cranks up will and desire. Remember what your mom used to tell you when you were tongue-tied and making no sense? "Use your words." Stating your intended goal as simply, clearly, and positively as you can manage really helps.

You already have plenty of voices in your head. Some may be telling you that you're fat, or that you'll never be good enough, or that you're going to fail at any sort of self-improvement. These are self-perpetuating hang-overs from childhood and have no bearing on your present conscious adult life and no place in your future. Drown out those doubting voices you inherited from others with positive affirmations in your own voice. Stand and deliver. It's high time for true talk. Say out loud that *Enough is enough, I am ready to be well. My health is my wealth. Today and every one of the rest of my days on this planet, I'm fighting to be healthy.* The principle of Will and Desire is only ever just a sentence away.

THE WORD

My Sistah Erykah Badu and I have known each other for more than a dozen years, ever since Erykah walked into Frank's Poetry Spot one night in 1996 when I was doing a spoken word performance. Turns out that even though we'd never before met when Erykah strolled in off the curb that night, she had just finished reading my mother's book *Heal Thyself.* It was also the same year that Erykah recorded *Baduizm* and "On and On." "A lot of amazing things were happening in that one year for me," she says, "a lot of noncoincidental things, things that were destined to, and that I started putting together.

"For me it's all about making sure that your willpower is good," Erykah said. "It's all in the choices that you make, the responsibility you take for the choices that you make, and the stamina you exert to get that energy out. The one important thing that we should always remember about the will is that it has to be exercised, like any other muscle. When you're lying in bed, the will is the thing saying, 'Get up now, go, go, go!' I think one of the most powerful things that you have is that thing that says, 'Okay, you're not gonna drink anymore, you're not gonna smoke anymore.' 'But I like it,' you think. But your will, that voice, says, 'You're not gonna do it because you can't. If you do, then the heart can't do its job. You're gonna mess up everyone's program.' The will is always talking to us. And it's up to us to focus and listen and be there for the will.

"Life is all about intent. It's either come in peace or leave in pieces. You should say anything that you feel is good, especially if the intent is good." But the gift of willful speech has its responsibilities, too. "I have a very dry, deadpan type of humor and some people don't get it," Erykah says. "It doesn't feel too good to them, you know what I mean? It can be threatening and also offensive, I believe. I'm from the South and we have a habit of talking about people in a joking way and it's funny, it's jokey but then it's kinda hurtful if someone would ever hear us. It's just a habit. You just have to experience the consequences of it, to know how to deal with it. After you've seen people react you must be able to forgive them and yourself.

"I've been all over this planet and I've seen so many people and so many things," Erykah tells me. "We are all one thing. There's nothing happening to you that's not happening to anyone else." There's courage in that connection, she said. "I see so many people becoming conscious. People are rising up everywhere and resisting occupation more and more and more. I see it becoming a way of life. More and more people are eating right and more and more people are having discussions that are at a higher place. More and more people are doing yoga and all of the higher arts and the healing arts. There's a quickening going on. I like that word, a quickening. I see it happening all over the planet."

PART II

The Five-Week Supa Power Plan

Putting the Words into Practice

Count all the calories and carbs you want—the simple truth is that fat is the inevitable by-product of eating toxic food and not getting enough exercise. Those cottage cheese puckers on your butt and thighs, the double and triple chin, arm wattles, saddlebags, paunches, and rolls don't just trash your self-esteem, they're part of an inevitable doomsday scenario for your heart, your joints, your liver, and other organs, taxed to the max dealing with the excess poundage and the overloading and undernourishing diet that makes it happen.

That also goes for the energy you need in order to face each day. A Toxitarian diet simply puts you through the wringer.

* Body pH
* Cells
* Brain
* Libido
* Stomach
* Liver
* Kidneys
* Colon
* Blood

* Heart
* Muscles
* Lungs
* Immune system
* Lymph system
* Skin
* Eyes
* Hair

Every one of these perfectly designed blessings of life is maxed out by consuming the wrong foods made of the wrong ingredients at the wrong times.

Augment that Toxitarian diet with a modern sedentary lifestyle built around the TV, car, and computer, and a self-defeating occasional program of exercise, and you have the perfect recipe for a low-power, high-weight, high-illness life.

My Five-Week Supa Power Plan is designed to help you rev up and slim down by:

* Detoxing—Phasing out foods with properties and ingredients that make you sick, tired, and overweight.
* Cleansing—Using the power of proper nutrition to combat and rinse out the harmful residue of Toxitarian eating.
* Nourishing—Giving your body a therapeutic dose of the ingredients and nutrients that make you live and look your best.
* Working In—Cleanse, sculpt, and strengthen by getting busy with your body from the inside out.

Detox

Over the course of the first Foundation Four weeks of the program, we'll adjust what it is you eat to reduce the impact of harmful, toxic ingredients and foods.

✗ Meat
✗ Dairy
✗ Sugar
✗ Processed foods
✗ Chemical food additives

These are all known killers. Rather than dump all that stuff at once, during the Foundation Four, we'll take it a week at a time.

WEEK ONE–SUPA FLEXITARIAN
During the first week we'll dial back on added sugar and take red meat (beef and pork) out of the Toxitarian diet.

WEEK TWO–SUPA VEGETARIAN
In Week Two, chicken and fish and the toxins they contain are out— vegetables, legumes, and whole grains take over, and 50 to 75 percent of that will be live food or lightly steamed, to take full advantage of the enzyme nutrition in live vegetables that recovering Toxitarians and Starchitarians don't get in their diets.

WEEK THREE–SUPA RAW FOOD VEGAN
Raw food packs a knockout punch of body cleansing and energizing enzymes that are destroyed when food is heated or processed. This week of raw food is a literally vital way to change the course of a body that's burdened by toxicity and fat.

WEEK FOUR–SUPA JUICE FAST
Concluding the Foundation Four weeks of the Supa Power Plan is a seven-day juice fast. When you confine all your nutritional intake to chlorophyll-rich vegetable and fruit juice sources, your natural body pH will come back into balance. Pampered by the antioxidant vitamins, minerals, enzymes, oxygen, soluble fiber, and water of green juices and fruit alone, and unburdened by Toxitarian additives, your cells and the

organs and systems they maintain get a deluxe spa treatment of powerful fueling and easy digestion. Think of it as taking The Remedy to the next level.

Cleansing

All five weeks of the Supa Power Plan ask you to increase your intake of water and of "broom foods"—fiber and water-rich produce and grains that ensure your colon is working at maximum efficiency and that you remain in cleansing mode 24/7, the way nature intended. All five weeks also incorporate specific Chlorophyllian vegetable juice recipes that target organ systems in need of cleansing from the symptoms of a Toxitarian or Starchitarian diet.

* **Monday:** The Kidney Cleanser to assist your renal system in its never-ending job of straining toxins and water out of fifty gallons of blood a day.
* **Tuesday:** The Liver Cleanser turns back the clock on liver-challenging eating and drinking habits.
* **Wednesday:** Blood Builder addresses your blood's need for the right combination of nutritive factors to stay healthily pumping throughout your body.
* **Thursday:** Lymphatic Flush—a well-earned respite for this vast and underappreciated system of infection-fighting cells flowing throughout our bodies.
* **Friday:** Respiratory Cleanser, in tandem with five weeks of little or no mucus-generating dairy poisons, helps you to make the most out of each new breath.
* **Saturday:** Immune Booster, a potent assist for autoimmune function.
* **Sunday:** Colon Cleanser sees to it that your lower intestine gets a clean slate for Monday.

WEEK FIVE—THE SUPA CAPSTONE OF WELLNESS

By the fifth week of the Power Plan, you'll have experienced the benefits of four different but parallel and positive approaches to a healthier, more energized lifestyle. How you feel will dictate where you go next. Quick cleanse with The Remedy? Go back to a modified Flexitarian lifestyle followed by a juice fast? By Week Five you'll know what these choices mean to you, to your level of energy, your peace of mind, the way you see yourself both in the mirror and in relation to your family and the larger community around you. After twenty-eight days of structured menus, Week Five is a solo flight that sets the tone for the future. For the final week of the plan and for every week after, the choice of how to live will be up to you.

The Five Week Supa Power Plan is not a diet to be slavishly followed and then abandoned. It's not a diet at all. It's a simple and unadulterated way to put the principles of holistic health to good use and to consciously detox, cleanse, restore energy and health, and fight fat through proper eating.

Seven Steps to Colon Health

The average Toxitarian carries between 5 and 10 pounds of impacted waste in his or her colon. An impacted colon can cause:

* Protruding abdomen
* Gas
* Headaches
* High blood pressure
* Parasites
* Skin conditions such as boils or eczema

I recommend doing one or two of following during a Remedy Supa Cleanse and over the course of the Five-Week Supa Power Plan. Anything less than a healthy bowel movement after every meal leaves room for improvement.

✓ Soak 2 tablespoons of flaxseeds overnight. Blend with one 8-ounce glass of apple or pear juice the next day and enjoy.

✓ Eat a bowl of raw or steamed okra, or mix raw or steamed okra into a soup or salad.
✓ Take a mild herbal laxative one to three times a week until your colon is regulated.
✓ Drink 8 glasses of warm water every day.
✓ Gently massage your abdomen twice a day from the right (yours) to left.
✓ Visit a colon therapist for a colonic or take a warm water enema. For a stronger effect you can add lemon or lime juice to the enema bag to relieve gas and mucus congestion in the colon.
✓ Elevate your legs against the wall in a 45-degree angle for five to ten minutes as you lie flat on your bed to improve the circulation in the colon.

THE TRUTH

Each day of the five weeks positions the largest and, except for the juice fast week, most protein-intensive meal at the center of the day to work with the body's natural daily solar rhythm, not against it. Our metabolism and digestion are governed by the sun's daily rise and fall, the same as every other cycle of life on earth. Our bodies are sluggish at sunup, build to a peak of energy and flow by midday, then start to power back down as the sun sets. Digestion and excretion are at their optimum performance level at midday and less active after the sun goes down and in the early morning hours.

We all know that when we sleep at night, our unconscious minds are working overtime to digest all the experiences and sensations we've had since the previous night's sleep. While you sleep, your digestive system is doing the same thing, but at a greatly reduced rate. Sending it off to dreamland with a full gut throws its schedule off big-time. When you have a starchy, meaty meal after dark or late at night, your overtaxed digestive system has to put in an all-nighter while you sleep. The morning after a wee-hours trip to the drive-thru will leave you dehydrated, headachy, groggy, and tired. Midnight snacking brings on a food hangover the next day, with many of the same symptoms as the kind of hangover you get from drinking too much booze.

"Duh" moment—breakfast means "break fast," right? When we awaken in the morning, we should be in a fasting state. That means a relatively empty stomach and, after a quick trip to the john once we're up, empty bowels. Feeding a recently awakened body that's just been reborn into the world a big, starchy, high-calorie, bacon and egg and toast and grits breakfast is a shock to the system. I don't care what any study of schoolkids in Iowa says: A big meal first thing in the day is cruel and unusual punishment for a body coming out of the deep.

For complete, holistic health, the traditional big breakfast, light lunch, and big dinner is out. A large lunch dominated by broom foods like protein-rich legumes, leafy vegetables, and whole grains needs to be the consciously and strictly observed central eating experience of your day. That's when you're best equipped to deal with the dietary heavy lifting. The spokes of that hub meal reach back to a light breakfast that doesn't give your still-awakening body the caloric waterboard treatment, and forward to a dinner that, like in most African, tropical, Mediterranean, and other warm climate cultures, is small and primarily fruits and vegetables.

The schedule for the Week One Flexitarian meals gives a good indication of how to work with the sun to maximize the Power Plan's cleanse and restoration:

Morning Surge: First thing when you wake up
Supa Breakfast: Between 6 and 9 A.M.
Midday Energizer: Anytime from one hour after breakfast up to one hour before lunch
Supa Lunch: Noon–1 P.M.
Afternoon Stabilizer: Anytime from one hour after lunch to one hour before dinner
Power Supper: 6–7 P.M.
Supa Snack: Anytime from an hour after dinner to one hour before bed

THE BODY

As the Remedy Five-Week Power Plan flushes, cleanses, and rejuvenates you through the food you eat, a weekly schedule of accompanying exercises will give you something to do with all that newfound energy.

Exercise benefits every single part of you:

✓ Increased breathing rate and pulse oxygenates the blood.
✓ Breathing fast and sweating more detoxifies.
✓ Vigorous motion improves the way food physically moves through your digestive tract and how the lymphatic system circulates infection-fighting lymph throughout the body.
✓ It aids in calcium and other nutrient absorption.
✓ It improves mood through the release of endorphins.
✓ Exercise improves clarity of thought, sleep, cholesterol and LDL levels, body pH, your body weight, and your sex drive!

All these things stabilize or improve when you work regular exercise into your life.

WHAT'S GOOD?

All Five Weeks of the Supa Power Plan includes fresh vegetable juices, which you will need to prepare at home using a mechanical juicer. Home juicers range from around $35 to several hundred. A top-of-the-line Norwalk cold-press juicer will set you back around $2,500. Still cheaper than a home dialysis machine, but who's got that kind of money? Here's the skinny on affordable juicer models.

Centrifugal

These juicers force the vegetables and fruit that you feed them against high-speed rotating blades. In a centrifugal juicer, a carrot gets pulverized by the blades and then flung against the wall of a whirling, filter-equipped drum. The drum separates the nutrient-dense ingredients from the fiber and pulp, holding it all together by letting the rich liquid pass through and out the juicer's spout.

Pros:

✓ Cheap
✓ Available at Walmart, Target, and just about everywhere else

Cons:

✗ Messy cleanup with some models
✗ Noisy
✗ Oxygenates juice and makes froth

In a centrifugal juicer, once the produce hits the blade, the fuse is lit. Using rotating blades and a centrifuge to break up a fruit or a vegetable puts a little heat and a lot of additional oxygen into the mix. That oxygen instantly goes to work breaking down all that amazing nutrition. If you need to store fresh juice, do it in as airtight a container as possible and fill the container to the top so that there's as little air in there with the juice as possible.

Masticating

A masticating juicer chops up produce at a slower speed more conducive to juice extraction.

Pros:

✓ Juices are less frothy, especially leafy greens, and retain more nutritive power when stored
✓ More versatile and durable

Cons:

✗ Pricey (anywhere from ninety bucks for a hand-cranked model to as much as two to three times that much for an electric)
✗ Require a little more prep work and juicing time than the zap-and-go centrifugal juicers

TRITURATING

These machines have a twin pair of slow-moving elongated gears that finely grind veggies and fruits nice and thoroughly. If you can afford one (they run from about 350 to 700 bucks, even more for a top-of-the-line Norwalk juicer, unfortunately), they're well worth owning.

Pros:

✓ Very-high-quality juice

Cons:

✗ High price

THE TRUTH

Since the Five-Week Supa Power Plan puts so much emphasis on produce, it's important to buy organic. In the United States, food that is certified organic was not grown using pesticides or chemical fertilizers.

One of the few positives about our ongoing diet epidemic is that the demand for organic fruits, vegetables, and grains is growing, and enlightened farmers are heeding the call. It's not a moment too soon. World food prices are skyrocketing as more countries emulate the American processed food diet. With locally grown organic staples, there's much less cost from the energy demands of distribution and the expense of marketing. So, even though most organic food costs more than its inorganic counterpart, when you buy organic, especially locally grown organic, you're making a small but necessary step in the direction of bailing out the rest of the world, while giving your cells a break.

American farmers began spraying fruits, vegetables, and grains with pesticides and growing them with artificial, chemical-laced fertilizers decades ago. It is absolute insanity what goes into our food as it's being grown. The EPA now approves 371 different pesticides for use on strawberries alone. And the history of the various studies, approvals, and banning of specific toxic pesticides is rife with bias and misinformation from the companies that develop and manufacture the stuff. Also, since pesticides wipe out weeds and vermin, they wipe out the animals that feed on them, and wreak havoc on the natural order of things.

Let me bring it into your hood and up to your doorstep: A 2006 study of two common agricultural pesticides conducted by scientists at Emory University in Atlanta found that putting a group of children with measurable quantities of both chemicals in their urine on a diet of organically grown food eliminated almost any trace of those toxins in the kids' urine in just fifteen days. Two weeks of eating the right food was all it took for those children to detox. All that they had to do was switch to organic.

WHAT'S GOOD?

Your kitchen is a sacred place. It's a cipher where you call the shots. In the interest of your health, you should seriously consider making some of the following substitutions before beginning the Five-Week Power Plan:

✗ Plastic bottles
✗ Plastic spatulas
✗ Plastic bowls
✗ Plastic colanders
✗ Plastic cutting board
✗ Aluminum cookware
✗ Nonstick-coating cookware

✓ Glass
✓ Stainless Steel
✓ Enamel
✓ Earthenware
✓ Bamboo
✓ Hardwood
✓ Cast iron
✓ Rolled iron

No nukes: A microwave oven is an amazing high-science way to quickly heat food. It is also the single most efficient way to kill enzymes, neuter nutritional content, and wipe out minerals and moisture in anything you put into your body after you nuke it. If you have a microwave, get rid of it. You shouldn't disrespect your food by irradiating it like it's a cancerous tumor. For the duration of The Remedy's Five-Week Supa Power Plan, your microwave is going to be a wall clock and nothing more.

Also, while you're throwing stuff out, consider this—your skin is the largest organ in your body. It breathes, consumes, transforms, and deals with everything that touches it on a highly intimate basis. If you really want to do right by your skin, it's important to put only food-grade products on it. Anything you apply to your skin winds up in you anyway, so never put anything on your skin that you wouldn't want to put in your mouth. Most body creams, lotions, and cosmetics are made with water, alcohol, mineral oil, petroleum products, and all kinds of nasty chemicals. If you don't want that stuff in you, don't put it on you. Send all the lotions and moisturizers in your medicine cabinet that aren't made of natural, nonchemical ingredients to your garbage bag and think about substituting products like Sheago cosmetics, or one of the other available food-grade brands.

THE WORD

Since Sade's 1984 multiplatinum album, *Diamond Life* (on which he co-wrote the songs and played guitar and saxophone), UK-born musician, producer, and songwriter Stuart Matthewman has crisscrossed the globe with Sade and the band. But his first visit to the United States (where he now lives) was an eye-opener.

"The first time I came here, I just thought the sizes of the portions were massive," he says. "Even if you go into a McDonald's in Europe, the portions of the food are smaller than they are at a McDonald's here in the United States. The French fries and the sodas are like half as big. The size of the portions here are just outrageous. Normally in England and Europe, when you order a sandwich, it's for you personally to eat there and then. It's not that you're going to share it or necessarily take it home and eat the rest of it another day. And people here tend to eat until they're full and satisfied, so to speak. Whereas I personally—and this was just the way I was brought up—tended to eat just until I wasn't hungry. I was always likely on the go. I hate the idea of eating and then collapsing in front of the TV. I've always just eaten enough to keep me going. More of a grazer, I guess."

THE TRUTH

Eating out in America is a risky proposition. Over the course of the Five-Week Supa Power Plan, try to limit your restaurant visits to places where you can get the kinds of foods represented in each week's menu. Of course, not every town has a raw food or vegan restaurant, and there's no guarantee that just because a restaurant is vegetarian, it's actually good in the first place. You just never know. When going out to eat, keep this in mind:

* Cuisines from Asian countries tend to have the healthiest options, as most Asian cuisines foreground the vegetables and background the meat.
* If your server or the counterperson can't tell you what's in a menu item, don't order it.
* If a sauce can't be left off or put on the side, don't order the menu item.
* Just because an item is listed as vegetarian or vegan doesn't mean that it's healthy. Many "vegetarian" menu items are just Starchitarian fare in disguise.

THE LOVE

We'll examine the remaining five principles over the five weeks of the Supa Power Plan. Going in, though, I want you to promise yourself one thing. Over the course of Power Plan, do not indulge in angry eating. Being tired is one thing, but if you're pissed off, depressed, anxious, scared, bugged out, or frustrated beyond your conscious ability to relieve, do not sit down to a regular meal until you're back on smoother emotional ground. When you consume food while in a state of emotional turmoil, you're almost guaranteed to relate to the taste, texture, and the ritual of a meal as a means of self-medication. Angry eating is unconscious eating. Food is fuel and food is life. It's not a Band-Aid or a distraction from emotional pain.

If mealtime arrives and you're angry, hurt, or freaked out emotionally, write down what led to that feeling in your notebook and describe where it's coming from. Then:

* Take a walk
* Get a massage
* Talk to someone you love and trust
* Stop talking to someone you hate and fear
* Turn off the phone, TV, or computer
* Go to the gym

Don't use food to change your mental weather.

Jot down the thoughts and memories and experiences that accompany your meals and meal preparation in your notebook. We want to spend part of the next thirty-five days exposing and defusing the triggers that cause self-medicating eating, when food is used as a drug, rather than as the fuel and healthful blessing that it is.

two

Week One—The Flexitarian

THE TRUTH

The biggest lie in the American diet is that you need meat, dairy, and other animal proteins in order to live. This tall tale gets retold generation after generation for two reasons:

1. Meat and dairy are a huge business.
2. We don't understand the true place that protein has in our diets.

Red meat simply doesn't do enough for us to earn a place on our plates. What human bodies primarily need to grow and thrive are:

* Oxygen
* Water
* Amino acids
* Enzymes
* Vitamins and minerals
* Fiber
* Carbohydrates
* Essential oils

MUST HAVES	BEEF/PORK	CHICKEN	FISH	DAIRY	PROCESSED GRAINS	WHOLE GRAINS	FRUIT	VEGETABLES
Oxygen	No	No	No	No	No	No	Yes	Yes
Water	No	No	No	No	No	No	Yes	Yes
Amino Acids	Yes	Yes	Yes	Yes	Yes	Yes	Yes	Yes
Enzymes	Yes	Yes	Yes	Yes	Yes	Yes	Yes	Yes
Vitamins and minerals	Yes	Yes	Yes	Yes	Yes	Yes	Yes	Yes
Fiber	No	No	No	No	No	Yes	Yes	Yes
Complex carbohy-drates	No	No	No	No	No	Yes	Yes	Yes
Essential oils	No	No	Yes	No	No	Yes	Yes	Yes

Fresh fruits and raw vegetables have all of those things in abundance. Red meat has only three. Yet for the majority of Americans it's the main event in the meal. The Week-One Flexitarian menu takes a page out of most traditional Asian cuisines and uses meat sparingly—like a garnish and not the star attraction.

Commercially raised red meat also contains a bunch of things that we don't need:

✗ Heavy metals, plastics, PCBs. and other industrial contaminates
✗ Pesticides—from sprayed feed grains
✗ Antibiotics/tranquilizers
✗ Genetic alterations—in both the animal flesh and in their feed
✗ High-acid pH
✗ A natural resistance to absorption and excretion in the human colon

MUST AVOIDS	BEEF/PORK	CHICKEN	FISH	DAIRY	PROCESS GRAINS	WHOLE GRAINS	INORGANIC PRODUCE	ORGANIC PRODUCE
Heavy metals/ PCBs	Yes	Yes	Yes	Yes	No	No	No	No
Pesticides	Yes	Yes	Yes	Yes	Yes	Yes	Yes	No
Growth hormones	Yes	Yes	Yes	Yes	No	No	No	No
Antibiotics/ tranquil- izers	Yes	Yes	Yes	Yes	No	No	No	No
GMO	Yes	Yes	Yes	Yes	Yes	Yes	Yes	No
Acid pH	Yes	Yes	Yes	Yes	Yes	No	No	No
Colon threat	Yes	Yes	Yes	Yes	Yes	No	No	No

WHAT'S GOOD?

For the first week of the Power Plan, the two red meat staples—

- ✗ Beef
- ✗ Pork

—are casualties of our journey to wellness. The only two permissible flesh foods for the first week are:

- ✓ Chicken—breast only, free-range if possible, no more than 4 ounces (about the size of a cassette tape) per serving.
- ✓ Fish—filet only, domestic farm raised or wild catch, also 4 ounces max.

Consuming fish brings up a toxicity issue all its own. According to a November 2008 article in the *New York Times*, the United Nations' Food and Agricultural Organization has concluded that "the maximum wild-capture fisheries potential from the world's oceans has probably been reached." A 2006 study, the *Times* says, "concluded that if current fishing practices continue, the world's major commercial stocks will collapse by 2048."

Holistic living makes some choices all too easy. With the world's oceans in environmental crisis, most fish have become too toxic to eat anyway. The following fish are too contaminated with land run-off chemicals and sea pollutants to eat:

- ✗ Cod
- ✗ Snapper
- ✗ Bluefish
- ✗ Swordfish
- ✗ Tuna
- ✗ Sole
- ✗ Mahi-mahi
- ✗ Pollock
- ✗ Channel catfish
- ✗ Porgy
- ✗ Orange Roughy
- ✗ Lake Trout
- ✗ Bonito
- ✗ Rockfish
- ✗ Mackerel

Add to that list:

- ✗ Crab
- ✗ Oysters
- ✗ Lobster

✗ Shrimp
✗ Clams
✗ Mussels

Even under natural conditions, shellfish feed on filth. They've been forbidden at my house for my whole life. Now that most shrimp and lobster is farm-raised overseas under extremely unsanitary conditions, shellfish are more out than ever.

Acceptable fish for the Flexitarian are:

✓ Flounder
✓ Haddock
✓ Domestic-farmed Trout
✓ Pacific Salmon

Transitioning Flexitarians should choose the bulk of their protein foods from legumes—the bean family. They're loaded with vital amino acids, minerals, and vitamins and, like fruit, vegetables, and whole grains, match their nutritive value with a healthy dose of fiber.

✓ Kidney beans
✓ Black beans
✓ Pinto beans
✓ Garbanzo beans/chickpeas
✓ Green, red, black, and brown lentils
✓ Split peas
✓ Black-eyed peas
✓ Soy beans
✓ Pigeon peas

THE TRUTH

There are three components that make fruits and vegetables the perfect foods.

1. High water content
2. High fiber content
3. High nutrition content

When I say "fiber" I'm talking about dietary fiber—any of a number of naturally occurring organic substances that don't digest in the body and that pass through us. Dietary fiber comes in two strains: soluble fiber, which mixes and dissolves in liquid, and insoluble fiber, which stays whole, rough, and ready even in water. Think of the two kinds of fiber as two kinds of brooms.

* **Insoluble fiber** is the bigger, coarser cleaner-upper: It keeps things smooth and keeps things moving and keeps intestinal pH on point.
* **Soluble fiber** does the detail work: It cozies up to fatty acids and toxins that need encouragement to exit, regulates digestion so that your blood sugar gets a full opportunity to make the most of what you've eaten, and works with bacteria in your colon to mine vitamin B12 from microorganisms within you.

Nutrient-wise, fruits and vegetables are loaded with healthy enzymes, vitamins, and minerals, and are the best-known source of two of the most talked-about aspects of nutrition today:

* Antioxidants
* Phytochemicals

One of the most miraculous relationships between food and body is the balance between the oxygen your blood and tissues thrive on and the antioxidant vitamins and minerals you're supposed to be consuming along with it. Pollution, pesticides, cigarette smoke, and even some of the body's own metabolic processes form unstable, destructive molecules called free radicals that use oxygen to break down and attack your cells. The natural, serene, *no problemo* countermeasure we literally bring to the table to combat free radicals are *antioxidants*.

Antioxidants are the sharp-eyed and discreet bouncers getting an annoying drunk away from our table and escorting him to the door of the club. When our plate is loaded with nutritious stuff like leafy green vegetables, the antioxidant vitamins, minerals, and enzymes in those foods naturally counter and slow the molecular destruction to our cells caused by free radicals. *Phytochemicals* are still being identified. They're a class of highly potent micronutrient free radicals that are in most dark-pigmented vegetables and fruits.

THE WORD

Melyssa Ford combines beauty with brains. Via her modeling work, her bestselling videos, her column in *Smooth Magazine,* and her duties as on-air host of Sirius Radio's *Hot Jamz,* Melyssa's voice, wit, and curves are known by millions. But the way the Toronto, Canada, native sees herself may surprise those picturing her pinup calendars. "I'm like a Clydesdale," she said recently when I asked hip-hop's "Jessica Rabbit" about her relationship with food. "I'm West Indian on my father's side and Russian and Norwegian on my mother's," she explained. "My genetics dictate that I can get big! I'm a clotheshorse, I love fashion, and sample sizes are really, really tiny. So I have to monitor my eating habits if I have a hope in hell of maintaining a small size. It takes a lot of dedication and it takes a lot of effort on my part to control my eating, 'cause I can eat like a football player. For real!

"For a large portion of my life, my relationship with food was a love-hate one," Melyssa said. "I looked at food as the enemy. I've always been very health-conscious and I've always known how to eat right, but knowing how to do it and *wanting* to do it are two very, very different things. I used to go through periods of time where I would try to starve or use thermagenic supplements in order to suppress my appetite."

Like just about everyone, Melyssa's tempestuous romance with what she eats began in childhood. "I was eight years old and I was sitting on my mom's bed and I was sitting cross-legged," she remembered. "If you have a big butt, when you sit cross-legged, your butt kinda spreads to the side. So I'm sitting cross-legged in my mom's room and I look down and I was like, 'Mom, what's that?' She said, 'That's your butt.' So then I was like, 'Well, why is it over there?' Mom said, 'I don't know.' So I asked her how to get rid of it and she said, 'Exercise.' She has no idea the damage that she caused on that day!" Melyssa laughed. "From that moment on, I promise you, I developed body dysmorphic disorder! I was trying to fight what I couldn't fight. I was born with an ass and it is an extremely large ass, but it is what it is. That's where my fascination and I guess obsession with food and my unhealthy attitude towards it started."

Thankfully, Melyssa's childhood curiosity matured into the habit of educating herself: "It made me seek out information on how to live a healthy lifestyle and how to eat and exercise properly." Being born in a nation with a national health system that promotes effective public health education didn't hurt. "In the supermarkets in Canada, it's almost like a party on Saturdays and Sundays," Melyssa said. "There are clowns making balloons for kids, there's cake being served. You can go down any aisle and there are taste tests of new products and stuff like that. But then the most interesting thing about supermarkets in Canada is the fact that you can also go down any single aisle and find pamphlets and brochures providing information on how to eat right and how to start living a healthy lifestyle, rather than just thinking *diet*. In Canada, healthy lifestyles and a healthy way of eating are heavily promoted."

This was not exactly the case when Melyssa arrived in the United

States. "When I came to the States almost eight years ago, I moved to Brooklyn. I went to the supermarket and was appalled on so many different levels," she recalled. "I mean, from the produce department on down, it was disgusting. I would sooner consume food in cans than try to pick up what they deemed fresh produce. And there was no information given on how to eat right.

"I guess I'm just fortunate because of where I was raised," Melyssa said. "And I've also always been thirsty to educate myself on things that I found myself curious about. In Canada, that information is so readily available to us, basically wherever we go. But in New York, it seems like unless you live on 63rd and Madison, you really don't have a chance of trying to educate yourself on how to eat right or change your eating habits or your health. If I had been raised in Brooklyn, I might not see a problem in consuming McDonald's three, four times a week. I might not see a problem in drinking soda instead of pure cranberry juice, pure orange juice, or even water. I might not see a problem with having potato chips as a snack versus some slices of apple and some reduced-fat peanut butter."

Her learning process continues. "I try and educate myself on foods that have certain healthful properties, that are known to prevent certain diseases, like broccoli, kale, really green vegetables, really red vegetables," she explained. "Foods that are vibrant in color seem to be so high in antioxidants that they ward off diseases and illnesses. So I try to make my diet as colorful as possible. I do eat a lot of fresh vegetables and fruit."

WHAT'S GOOD?

Generally then, the greener, orange-er, or redder a vegetable is, the better it is for you. Top-tier healthy vegetables include:

- ✓ Spinach
- ✓ Kale
- ✓ Swiss chard

- ✓ Broccoli
- ✓ Okra
- ✓ Cabbage
- ✓ Mustard greens
- ✓ Brussels sprouts
- ✓ Romaine lettuce
- ✓ Arugula
- ✓ Green beans
- ✓ Green peas
- ✓ Sea veggies like nori and other ocean greens
- ✓ Beets
- ✓ Carrots
- ✓ Sweet potatoes/yams
- ✓ Cauliflower
- ✓ Red, green, and yellow peppers
- ✓ Squash
- ✓ Mung, alfalfa, and soybean sprouts

Fruit also advertises its own health properties with deep colors. Eat any of the following knowing that you're nourishing yourself with food perfection:

- ✓ Blueberries
- ✓ Apples
- ✓ Bananas
- ✓ Oranges
- ✓ Lemons
- ✓ Limes
- ✓ Grapefruit
- ✓ Red and green grapes and brown and gold raisins
- ✓ Plums and prunes
- ✓ Pears
- ✓ Cantaloupe

✓ Watermelon
✓ Papaya
✓ Raspberries
✓ Strawberries
✓ Pineapple
✓ Kiwi

THE TRUTH

The American grain of choice is of course wheat, which—in its natural state—is a three-part harmony of:

1. The bran (the part with the fiber in it)
2. The germ (the part with most of the nutrition in it)
3. The endosperm (the part with the starchy simple carbohydrates in it)

But on the American plan, in order to save cooking time, the whole-wheat kernel has the hull, bran, and everything else in it milled away until only the starchy parts remain. That starchy ghost food then gets mixed with B vitamins and minerals (mostly iron) that for the most part would still be there if the wheat hadn't been given an industrial beating in the first place. White flour and white-flour products spike blood sugar and help gum up the lower intestine. To invite enriched white flour or enriched, processed grain products of any kind into your kitchen cipher is a waste of shelf space and of your body's digestive skills.

WHAT'S GOOD?

Grains need to be judged by their fiber content. If it's whole grain and unprocessed, it's in. Any whole-grain food, pasta, pilaf, bread, muffin, or other item is okay, as long as it wasn't made with enough sugar and additives to make it stealth candy.

Beware of heavily processed fake "whole grain" foods like whole-wheat Wonder Bread and "multigrain" snacks like Sun Chips, which put back small amounts of insoluble fiber in what's otherwise a starch-o-centric, additive-heavy laboratory creation. If the first word in a grain product's list of ingredients isn't "whole," then it isn't for you. And you can forget about most breakfast cereals. Unprocessed oatmeal (check the ingredients—if it's more than whole oats, it's not for eating) and organically grown, additive-free box cereals like Kashi get the thumbs-up, but even seemingly innocent breakfast cereals like Cheerios and cornflakes are secret sugar crack dealers and can contain hydrogenated oils, modified food starch, and preservatives galore. Just read the label.

Replace white flour with whole-grain flour and replace white-flour pasta, bread, crackers, etc., with real-deal brands and products.

Bionaturae's or Eden Foods's buckwheat pasta and DeBoles's artichoke flour, corn, and whole-wheat pasta are available at more and more supermarkets. These get the thumbs-up, too: any brand of 100-percent whole-wheat bread that's not made with enriched flour, hydrogenated oils, and corn syrup (most are—read the label and look for those words); simple whole-grain pita bread (again, read the label—anything more than whole wheat flour, yeast, water, and salt is out); and crackers from companies like Ak-Mak, Ryvita, and Wasa.

These are the amber waves to look for, try out, and experiment with:

✓ Whole wheat
✓ Bulgur wheat
✓ Spelt
✓ Kamut
✓ Buckwheat (or kasha)
✓ Rye flour
✓ Couscous
✓ Steel-cut oats

✓ Corn
✓ Brown rice
✓ Basmati
✓ Wild rice
✓ Amaranth
✓ Quinoa
✓ Millet
✓ Barley

THE WORD

Painter and poet Leroy Campbell has been part of my family's cipher for so long that I've called him Uncle my entire life. Leroy Campbell's art—like his celebrated Neck Bone series of canvasses—blend colors, shapes, and faces that evoke his African heritage and Southern childhood and the Black American experience in life, history, and music.

"I'm from Charleston, South Carolina, and I was born and raised on corn bread and black-eyed peas," Leroy explained. "We were called Gullah and Geechee people. We are descendents of slaves that came from West Africa and the Caribbean. My family and everyone around us, we had a variety of foods. The main staples were the greens, the vegetable. We had nuts and beans, grains, corn; we ate pork, fish, chicken, and turkey. We never just hung on one food. At that time pesticides weren't used on everything. And we didn't support fast food. We lived in a community where a lot of people came up from humble beginnings. People would consider us poor, but we cooked our food, we took the time to shop for our food. Some of us would go to the farmers' fruit stand or we'd go out to the country. Other times the farmers would come with their wagons. The fruit and vegetable man would come to the neighborhood maybe two or three times a week, and the fish man, all with fresh picked goods, all with fresh food."

"In Southern life, there's a tradition of passing along our food ways,"

Leroy explained. "Corn and the sweet potatoes, mixing and matching, putting that together with the tomatoes and spices, all that stuff comes about from having a Southern diet influenced by African and Caribbean heritage and my people's contact with Native Americans. For instance, red rice with green peppers and onions—that's the same thing as jollof rice in Senegal. We have a dish called hopping john, which in a Jamaican restaurant is peas and rice."

Leroy Campbell sees the healthy lifestyle he lives now as keeping the promise of his family's traditions. "The rest of my family, they'll say 'Your mama and your granddaddy lived to be eighty years old, your aunt lived to be ninety—they didn't die from the food they eat!' But at the time Grandma and Grandma were growing up, they were eating organic food. They grew up on their mother's milk. They were breast-fed, so their immune system was strong. By the time the eighties and the nineties came in, my elders were eating too much pork and they weren't working out. There are still people in my family that think, 'Well, I'm just gonna eat and die.' They don't realize you can live longer."

THE TRUTH

During the 1980s, Americans began to eat more sugar than ever before—and more than in any other country in history. Current estimates indicate that Americans do up between two and three pounds of sugar per week—each! That's an annual per capita consumption of 135 pounds a head. The huge spike in American sugar consumption has as much to do with the main course as it does with snacks and desserts. Refined sugar made from sugarcane, corn, and sugar beets has been smuggled into almost every processed food on the supermarket shelf. Cookies, candy, and soda are one thing, but sugar can turn up in staggeringly high quantities in:

X Mayonnaise
X Ketchup

X Spaghetti sauce

X Hot dogs

X Cured meats

X Canned vegetables

X Canned beans

X Soups

X Bread

X Pasta

X Microwavable meals

Read the label.

X High fructose corn syrup

X Sucrose

X Fructose

X Dextrose

X Maltodextrin (or "malodextrin")

X Maple syrup

X Molasses

X Honey

X Turbinado

X Brown sugar

X Rice syrup

X Amazake

X Carob powder

X Evaporated cane juice

All mean the same thing: sugar. And cutting sugar out merely on the basis of tooth decay, weight gain, or even Type II diabetes is selling a really toxic food trend way short. Addiction breeds denial, but you have to give it up to the truth—we are a nation strung out on sugar crack. Check this headline in the November 10, 2007, *L.A. Times:* "In a study, rats overwhelmingly prefer sweetened water to cocaine, even those already hooked on the drug." The article goes on to say that a team of French scientists offered lab rats the choice of a bump of coke dissolved in water, or a dose of sweetness-laced water. The rats went for the candy over the blow every time. "Intense sweetness is more rewarding to the rats than cocaine," one of the authors of the study said. It's the same with humans. Sugar crack dangerously elevates levels of dopamine and serotonin in the brain just like any other addictive drug, and drills a permanent craving into our minds that's nearly impossible to shake. Studies of infants and newborns have shown that once a kid's brain gets a taste of sugar crack, the kid will prefer to drink any sweetened beverage over water from then on.

First and foremost, sugar has extremely acid pH. There is absolutely no way your body can achieve homeostasis on the twenty to forty teaspoons of sugar unwittingly consumed per day by most Americans in sweetened processed foods and soda. Also refined, smuggled sugar messes with the body's glycemic index, the measure of how much of the correctly broken down nutrient sugar glycogen belongs in the bloodstream. The cells that make up your organs, muscles, bones, brain, and everything else are supposed to receive a nice even flow of the real sweet stuff that you naturally refine from complex carbohydrates and nutritious food sources. When you bomb yourself with all that additional, totally redundant simple sugar, the resulting spiking and plunging blood sugar levels dog your pancreas, the organ that produces insulin to metabolize glycogen, and puts you through mood swings, depression, and constant shock treatment.

Ongoing studies are finding the smoking gun of sugar crack behind:

* Alzheimer's disease and dementia
* Yeast infections
* Poor calcium absorption and osteoporosis
* Muscle and cartilage damage
* Suppressed immune system function

WHAT'S GOOD?

Common sugar substitutes like NutraSweet, Sucralose, and Aspartame are as suspect as the real thing. The only acceptable sugar replacements are:

✓ Stevia
✓ Agave nectar

—both of which are available online or at health food stores. For the beginning Flexitarian, substitution is the key.

For a milk substitute:

✓ Soy milk
✓ Almond milk
✓ Sesame milk

Soy milk is naturally low in cholesterol, but not necessarily low in fat, and can carry a lot of sugar in it. Read that label. If you want low-fat, unsweetened soy milk, make sure that's what you're buying. Rice milk tends to be more watery than soy milk, so as a straight swap out for cow's milk, it makes more sense to start with soy. Almond and sesame milk can be difficult to find, but they're worth seeking out. Also, almond milk, which is rich in vitamin E and has an appropriately nutty taste, is pretty easy to make.

For a cheese substitute:

✓ Soy cheese
✓ Grated tofu

For butter and corn oil margarine:

✓ Safflower margarine
✓ Olive oil

For chicken and beef soup stock and bouillon substitute:

✓ Vegetable stock and broth

For bleached white flour:

✓ Whole-wheat flour
✓ Buckwheat flour
✓ Barley flour
✓ Soy flour

For the Flexitarian week, we're substituting small amounts of lean, skinless chicken and fish for red meat. Other protein foods that can fill in for flesh include:

✓ Tofu
✓ Tempeh
✓ TVP
✓ Seitan

The other key food item for transitioning Flexitarians looking to cut down on meat-diet toxicity are prepared meat substitutes like veggie burgers and tofu dogs. But our processing-crazy food industry has seen to it that some veggie patties are better suited to Starchitarian diets.

✗ Morningstar Farms
✗ Boca Burgers
✗ Gardenburger

✗ Health Valley
✗ Subway's Veggie Patty

All of these contain various dairy ingredients like caseine or egg whites, plus preservatives, food colorings, and/or excess salt. Also, unless it says "non-GMO" somewhere on a product's container, it's almost a sure bet that the corporate soy-based veggie meats are made with genetically altered soybeans.

Yves's and Tofurky's meat substitute creations are among the leading brands that are non-GMO and take a sensible approach to salt and additive content. Ultimately it's up to you to read the label—if you can't pronounce, or don't recognize an ingredient, don't buy and eat the food that it's in.

Toxitarian or Starchitarian, the rule is the same: Use processed fake-meat foods the same way we are using chicken and fish in week one—as a garnish on a meal dominated by greens and whole grains, not the center of attention jammed between two white-flour rolls. Eating a veggie burger is substantially better for you than a cow burger, but living off of tofu pups, carrot chips, and frozen onion rings is not going to get your pH between the goal posts and help you cleanse and purify your body.

THE PLAN

WEEK 1 MONDAY

Morning Surge
1 teaspoon of Supa Mega Greens formula in pure apple juice

Supa Breakfast
2 slices of soy bacon, 1–2 slices of soy sausage, sliced pear, 6 ounces of granola with soy milk

Midday Energizer
Kidney Cleanser Supa Juice:
½ cup (about one handful) arugula, 2 celery stalks, ½ cup Swiss chard,

and 8–16 oz. of water. Add one juiced slice of apple to taste if necessary.

Arugula is more than just a slightly exotic salad addition. Its dark green leaves (an indication as always that a vegetable is rich in chlorophyll) and moist, peppery stalks contain beta carotene, potassium, and an abundance of chlorophyll and chemical compounds called glucosinolates that taken in low doses help to stimulate your body's own detoxifying process. Combining this with celery's own high potassium content and phytochemical compounds called coumarins, which help stimulate white blood cells and ease blood pressure, and Swiss chard, another slightly bitter green loaded with potassium and a treasure trove of other vitamins, the Kidney Cleanser gives your renal system a much-needed boost.

Supa Lunch

4 oz. broiled free-range organic white meat chicken
1 cup steamed millet
6–12 oz. steamed broccoli

Afternoon Stabilizer

Kidney Cleanser Supa Juice

Power Dinner

Chickpea soup with okra and scallions (*see page 189 for recipe*)
Tabouli salad with raw spinach and yellow peppers

Supa Snack

Raspberries w/apple slices

WEEK 1 TUESDAY

Morning Surge

2 tsp. of Supa Mega Greens in pear juice

Supa Breakfast

½ cup soaked almonds with raisins—leaving natural, unroasted almonds in water the night before awakens their sprouting vitality by breakfast time the next day. Drain them and serve them with raisins.
1 cup whole oats cereal
Sliced pear

Midday Energizer

Liver Cleanser Supa Juice:
½ a medium-sized beet and two artichokes blended with 8–16 oz. of water and a slice of apple to taste if you need it.

Beets romance your liver's natural detoxifying function almost better than any other food. As a beginning Flexitarian, you'll want to take it easy with beet power, as beets stimulate the liver and bowels pretty aggressively (and very healthily). That purging action catches newbies by surprise sometimes. A juiced artichoke is rich in choleretics, a group of natural chemical compounds that stimulate bile transmission from the liver to the gallbladder. This juice is a very potent and vital assist for your liver in its mission to detoxify you naturally, and a great way to finally do it a favor with the right food after overtaxing it with the wrong food.

Supa Lunch

Oven-steamed fish (*see page 190 for recipe*)
Brown rice (prepare 1 cup, enough for two meals)
Steamed string beans

Afternoon Stabilizer

Liver Cleanser Supa Juice

Power Dinner

Black beans and brown rice (the extra you made at lunch)
Green salad with Chef Ali's dressing (*see page 199 for recipe*)

Supa Snack

Blueberries with pear slices

WEEK 1 WEDNESDAY

Morning Surge

2 tsp. Supa Mega Greens with real cranberry juice and apple juice

Supa Breakfast

Soy sausage
Blueberry oat muffin
4 sliced strawberries

Midday Energizer

Blood Builder Supa Juice:
1 parsnip, ½ cup Swiss chard, ½ cup beet greens, 8–16 oz. water

Parsnips help to balance blood sugar and stimulate blood cell growth. Chard with beet greens are an intense combination of iron sources to help fatigued blood get back up to strength.

Supa Lunch

Tuna in water, with black pepper veggie mayonnaise and arugula, alfalfa sprouts, and red peppers in a pita

Afternoon Stabilizer

Blood Builder Supa Juice

Power Dinner

Kidney, black bean, okra, and tomato stew (*see page 191 for recipe*)
Steamed cauliflower

Supa Snack

Unsalted air-popped popcorn with herb seasoning
Juice of half a lemon mixed with 8 oz. warm water

WEEK 1 THURSDAY

Morning Surge

2 tsp. Supa Mega Greens in 8–16 oz. grapefruit juice

Supa Breakfast

Granola or other organic, unsweetned cereal, with ½ cup of walnuts and rice milk
Sliced peaches

Midday Energizer

Lymphatic Flush Supa Juice:
2 red radishes, 1 small-to-medium cucumber, ½ cup broccoli with 8–16 oz. of water and a slice of apple if you have to.

Your lymphatic system takes a lot of punishment in the modern world. While shepherding fatty acids to your bloodstream, and manufacturing and distributing antibodies, your lymph nodes, clustered in your neck, groin, chest, and elsewhere throughout your body, are constantly attacking diseased and potentially cancerous cells. The combination of red radish's vitamin C and potassium boost, cucumber's silica content, and broccoli's phytochemicals helps your lymph system to refresh itself.

Supa Lunch

Oven-steamed Salmon (*see page 190 for recipe*)
Toasted pita
Tossed salad

Afternoon Stabilizer

Lymphatic Flush Supa Juice

Power Dinner

Steamed carrots, peas, and cabbage
1 cup of millet

Supa Snack

2 sliced oranges with pineapple chunks

WEEK 1 FRIDAY

Morning Surge

2 tsp. Supa Mega Green in orange juice

Supa Breakfast

½ grapefruit
½ cup steamed tofu
1 slice whole-wheat toast with almond butter

Midday Energizer

Respiratory Cleanser Supa Juice:
2 scallions, 2 red radishes, 8–16 oz. water, apple slice if
desired
     The scallion and red radish combination stimulates the sinuses and
helps expel sputum and phlegm. It's a great antidote to the respiratory
symptoms of dairy toxicity.

Supa Lunch

Curry Mock Chicken Salad on a bed of salad greens (*see page 191 for
recipe*)

Afternoon Stabilizer

Respiratory Cleaning Supa Juice

Power Dinner

"Beef" TVP Stew Beans (*see page 192 for recipe*)

Supa Snack

Apple, pear, and berry smoothie

WEEK 1 SATURDAY

Morning Surge
2 teaspoons Supa Mega Greens in 8–16 oz. blackberry juice

Supa Breakfast
Papaya slices
Oatmeal topped with blueberries
or
Blueberry Buckwheat Pancakes (*see page 193 for recipe*)

Midday Energizer
Immune Booster Supa Juice:
3 large leaves of dandelion greens, 3 large chicory leaves, juice of one whole lemon, ½ turnip, 8–16 oz. water, juiced, with apple slice if desired.

    The milky white sap of dandelion and chicory greens is loaded with vitamins and minerals and laced with taraxacin, a chemical compound that acts as a mild diuretic. Along with lemon juice, dandelion greens and chicory leaves help to drain toxins that weigh down immune function and restore and preserve pH.

Supa Lunch
Chef Ali's Home Style Signature BBQ Tofu (*see page 194 for recipe*) and salad

Afternoon Stabilizer
Immune Booster Supa Juice

Power Dinner
Bulgur Wheat (*see page 202 for recipe*) and spinach

Supa Snack
Apple slice with peanut butter

WEEK 1 SUNDAY

Morning Surge
2 tsp. Supa Mega Greens with papaya juice

Supa Breakfast
Sliced peaches
Cracked wheat cereal with 2 cups hulled sunflower seeds

Midday Energizer

Colon Cleanser Supa Juice:
2 leaves of dandelion greens, juice of ½ lemon—a more potent dose
of dandelion's one-two punch of intense nutrition with modest diuretic
properties targeted at the colon.

Supa Lunch

Tofurky "sausage" (sweet or hot) with okra
Organic sweet potatoes
Garden Greens salad (*see page 196 for recipe*)
Vegan Corn Bread (*see page 195 for recipe*)

Afternoon Stabilizer

Colon Cleanser Supa Juice

Power Dinner

Black-eyed peas, okra, and seaweed salad

Supa Snack

2 sectioned tangerines topped with raw coconut

THE BODY

The Remedy Five-Week Supa Power Plan Work-In

As the Remedy Five-Week Supa Power Plan flushes, cleanses, and rejuvenates you through the food you eat, these accompanying exercises will
give you something to do with all that energy.

Exercise benefits every single part of you. Increased breathing rates
and sweating help you to detox and strengthen your lungs. Increased
pulse oxygenates the blood, helps the liver and kidneys to do their jobs
better, and safeguards the heart. The motion of vigorous exercise improves motility (the movement of food and waste through your intestines) and digestion, and helps the lymphatic system increase its own
circulation of lymph throughout the body.

* Calcium and other nutrient absorption
* Mood
* Clarity of thought
* Sleep
* Cholesterol
* Sex drive
* Body weight

The benefits of regular exercise are simply too dramatic and too numerous—don't cheat yourself out of them.

The Remedy Power Plan Exercise regime starts with stretches to limber up your body so you can do the program safely, then incorporates body-sculpting strength training and pulse-pumping cardio work, and eventually combines all three. It's up to you to modify or change the program as you see and feel fit.

A few basic principles:

EVERYTHING WORKS TOGETHER.

When stretching, strength training, or doing cardio, remember that no one muscle or organ is doing all the work. The human body works two or more major muscle groups together to perform whatever physical task is at hand. Pulling toward you with your arms engages biceps (the "make a muscle" muscle on the front of your upper arm), shoulder muscles, and back muscles together. Pushing away uses triceps (the muscle under the back of your upper arm), chest, and shoulders. Standing up and sitting down engages quads (front of thigh), hamstrings (back of thigh), calves, and glutes (your butt muscles).

IT'S A TWO-WAY STREET.

When body sculpting (with or without weights), always remember to do the work in both directions. An overhead military shoulder press is only 50 percent effective if you give it all you have going, but your arm floats back down again after you're up. Though an exercise may concentrate on a specific motion or muscle, there are always more parts of you in play when you're working out.

DON'T FORCE IT.
Whether stretching, warming up, working out, or cooling down, push yourself only if it feels right, not because you feel like you're supposed to or that you have to in order to get results.

LISTEN TO YOUR BODY.
If it's singing, hit it! If you're sore, stiff, in pain, or out of sorts, dial back on the effort accordingly.

KEEP IT FUN!
Play music. Huff, puff, yell out loud if you want to! Just make sure that improving your health and appearance through exercise stays engaging and relevant for you.

BREATHE.
The key to a good, healthy workout is to breathe. Inhale deeply and exhale fully at all times. Time your exhale with the part of any strength-training exercise that requires the most effort (the push away from the wall or floor in a pushup, the standing upward motion in a squat). If you're short of breath, you're short of oxygen, and if you're short of oxygen, your muscles and blood aren't getting what they need to strengthen, tone, and grow.

DRINK WATER.
Drink water throughout any workout. It's the other key to fitness success. Flushing through sitting and breathing while working out can go to the next level only if you're hydrated.

WEEK ONE

Week One of the Power Plan Work-In begins as every individual work-in should begin—with breathing and stretches.

* Stretches should be done before (Warm-Up Stretch) and after (Cool-Down Stretch) every workout.
* Hold each stretch for 10 to 20 seconds ("one Mississippi, two Mississippi . . .") as a way to relax, warm up, and prepare the muscles to work.
* Hold for 20–30 seconds when cooling down after a workout to increase flexibility.
* Breathe deeply during the stretch and line up your exhalation with the deepest part of the stretch motion. Use the breath to control and deepen the stretch. If you wish to deepen and extend the movement, back off a little while inhaling, then take the stretch a little deeper while exhaling.
* NEVER force a stretch. You want to feel the movement extending and loosening up the muscle, not putting undue stress upon it.
* Stretching is sensual—a love embrace for your body, so do it with feeling, tenderness, and care.

Day 1

Breathing

Meditative Breath

Lie on your back with your arms relaxed by your sides and your legs lying out naturally. Relax and close your eyes. Gently breathe in through your nose, bringing the breath deep into your belly and allowing your lungs to fill. Hold for three seconds, then exhale through your mouth. Keep breathing and stay in this position for about five minutes. Think about the task at hand and visualize a successful result.

Warm-Up Stretch

Abdominal Stretch I

Remain flat on your back on the floor with your legs extended naturally and bring your arms overhead, resting them on the ground as if making a snow angel. Slowly pull your arms and legs away from your torso as if you were trying to make yourself taller.

Abdominal Stretch II

Gently bring your knees into your chest, placing your hands on your shins as you do. Holding the crouch, using your hands to stabilize, gently rotate your bent knees in a circular motions to the right and to the left.

Hamstring/Glute/Hip Stretch I

Lie on your back on the floor or mat with your knees bent and the soles of your feet on the floor. Inhale and then slowly exhale as you straighten your right leg and slowly bring it up toward your body, grasping it behind either the quad or the shin with your hands. Keep bringing it toward you until you feel the stretch in the back of your leg. Breathe normally and rotate your raised ankle first in one direction, then the other. Slowly let your leg return to the start position and repeat with the other leg.

Hamstring/Glute/Hip Stretch II

Lying on your back on the floor, pull your knees into your chest. Clasp your hands under your knees (between knees and hamstrings) and gently press your lower back and hips into the floor.

Hamstring/Glute/Hip Stretch III

Starting in Hamstring/Glute/Hip Stretch II position, straighten the right leg and bring it to the floor while pulling the left knee into your chest, feeling a stretch in your left hip. To enhance the stretch, GENTLY bring the left knee across the body and rest it on the floor on the right. Switch legs.

Marching Orders

Feet center, march in place lifting your knees as high as they'll comfortably go and pumping your arms as though you were running eight times, then eight more times with your feet shoulder width apart. Take deep, full breaths throughout.

Feet center, arms out to your sides, march in place four more times with your arms together over your head as you go.

Feet wide, march in place four more times, bringing your arms out and overhead.

Cool-Down Stretch

Hamstring/Glute/Hip Stretch I, II, and III

Day 2

Breathing

Meditative Breath

Warm-Up Stretch

Abdominal Stretch I and II

Abs

Basic Crunches

Lie on your back on an exercise mat or towel on the floor with your knees bent and the soles of your feet on the floor. Place your hands behind your head just above the neck and gently cradle head and neck. Tighten your abdominal muscles, and imagine you are bringing your belly button and spine together, allowing your shoulders and upper body to roll forward to compensate. With your lower back remaining glued to the floor, your eyes looking past your knees, take a deep breath and, as you exhale, contract your abs and, using your hands on your neck as a guide, bring your shoulders a few inches off the floor, holding the contraction for a few seconds while taking a breath. In the same controlled motion, lower your upper body back to the floor while exhaling. Make sure to keep your back, head, and neck aligned throughout the motion. Your chin should not be on your chest (imagine you have an orange under your chin and leave that amount of space) and your hands should NOT pull or tug at your head and neck.

Do three sets (a grouping of the same exercise done multiple times in sequence) of eight repetitions (reps—the number of times you do the given exercise in a set) resting thirty seconds between sets.

Cool-Down Stretch

Abdominal Stretch I and II

Kneeling Lower-Back Stretch

Kneel on the floor with knees almost shoulder-width apart, your hands on the front of your thighs (quads) for support. Inhale and then, while tightening your abs, exhale and gently arch your back into a cat stretch. Inhale and flatten your back to the start position.

Repeat *Abdominal Stretch I.*

Day 3

Warm-Up Stretch

Lunge Stretch

Kneel on the floor. Keeping your left knee on the floor, bring your right knee forward so that your right foot is flat on the floor and your knee is at a right angle to the floor. Make sure that your right knee is directly above your right ankle, and not forward over the toe. Inhale and slowly and gently press forward as you exhale, feeling the stretch in your right quad and hip flexor (the big tendon running from the top of your thigh into your hip). Do not overstretch. Switch legs.

Hamstring/Glute/Hip Stretch I, II, III

Cardio

Marching Orders

Sixteen times with arms bent, feet center; sixteen times with arms bent, feet wide.

Sixteen times feet center, arms out to your sides and up overhead.

Sixteen times feet shoulder-width apart, bringing your arms together over your head as you go.

Legs

Squats

Start with feet shoulder-width apart, keeping your back straight and your knees stable (bent, but not moving forward) and slowly lower your butt as though you are going to sit in a chair (use a sturdy chair underneath you if you are worried that you might fall), working to get your hamstrings parallel to the floor, then slowly come back up to standing. Make sure your knees do not come forward over your toes. Three sets of eight, resting for thirty seconds in between each.

Cool-Down Stretch

Lunge Stretch
Hamstring/Glute/Hip Stretch I, II, and III

Day 4

Warm-Up Stretch

Abdominal Stretch I and II
Hamstring/Glute/Hip Stretch II
Lower-Back Stretch

Standing with legs shoulder-width apart, bring your hands to your butt cheeks for support. Inhale then exhale, tightening your abs, and slowly and gently arch your back into a cat stretch until you feel the muscles in your lower back. Gently flatten your back into starting position, then repeat.

Abs

Basic Crunches, three sets of eight

Lower Back

Lower-Back Extensions

Lie facedown, placing your palms on the floor (or mat) with your forehead resting on the back of your hands. Inhale. Slowly exhale and, using your contracted abs as a focus, slowly lift your arms and upper body a few inches off the ground, then lower again. Three times should do it for now.

Lower-Back Stretch

Cool-Down Stretch

Abdominal Stretch I and II

Hamstring/Glute/Hip Stretch I, II, and III

Day 5

Warm-Up Stretch

Lunge Stretch

Hamstring/Glute/Hip Stretch I, II, and III

Cardio

Marching Orders

Legs

Squats

Lunges

Stand with your feet shoulder-width apart. Step forward with the right leg, heel first. Keep most of your weight on your heel until you move forward, back leg to front, enough that your right leg is at a right angle, right thigh nearly parallel to the floor. Check that your right knee is directly over the ankle, not ahead of it, and that it remains that way. Continue to come down on your right thigh until your left knee is close to, but not all the way to, the ground. Power your right leg back up using your right heel and return to the starting position. Switch legs. Repeat two sets of eight on each side.

Cool-Down Stretch

Lunge Stretch

Quad Stretch (Standing)

Abdominal Stretch I and II

Hamstring/Glute/Hip Stretch I, II, and III

Day 6

Warm-Up Stretch

Biceps Stretch

Standing with feet shoulder-width apart, bring your arms out to your sides and slightly behind you, palms up, fingers gently outstretched. Breathe evenly. Slowly rotate your palms backward until your thumbs are pointing to the back wall, and you feel a gentle stretch across the front of your upper arm. Reverse direction until you feel the stretch again. Breathe through and don't force the stretch.

Triceps Stretch

Standing with feet shoulder-width apart, place your left fingertips on your bent right elbow. Breathe evenly and, using your left hand to stabilize and guide, draw your right elbow back and up past your ear until it's alongside your head or as far as it will comfortably go in that direction, with your right hand and forearm loosely pointing down your back. Use the left hand to gently press the right elbow until you feel a stretch in the underside of your right arm. Switch sides.

Shoulder Stretch

Standing with feet shoulder-width apart, hold your right arm out to the side. Without moving your torso, draw your right arm in front of you and bring your left arm to meet it, placing your left hand on the outside of your upper right arm (between shoulder and elbow), gently clasping with your left hand and using it to bring your right arm across your chest until you feel a gentle stretch in your right shoulder. Breathe into the stretch and do not force it or hunch your shoulders. Switch sides and repeat.

Chest Stretch

Standing with feet shoulder-width apart, gently clasp your hands behind your back, keeping your arms straight (without locking your elbows) and your chest high. Gently lift your clasped hands toward the ceiling until you feel a stretch in your chest and shoulders.

Upper-Back Stretch

Standing with feet shoulder-width apart, clasp your hands in front of you, palm of right hand over back of left, let your chin drop to your chest, and round your back. Gently press forward, feeling a stretch in your upper back and the backs of your shoulders. Still stretching, slowly bring your arms to the left side until you feel a gentle stretch in the right side of your back, then bring your arms back to center. Release and switch left hand over right, drop your chin, round your back, and bring arms to the right side of the room and back to center. Release. Breathe evenly throughout.

Arms

Biceps Curls

Stand with feet shoulder-width apart, arms fully extended in front of the body, palms facing out, and elbows supported gently by your waist. Take a breath and exhale as you bend your elbows, keeping them still touching your waist, and slowly curl your forearms up as far as they'll go toward your biceps, then slowly lower them until the arms are fully extended again. Three sets of eight reps.

Biceps Stretch

Triceps Kickback

Standing with legs together and knees slightly bent, lean forward at a 45-degree angle and put your arms by your side with your elbows bent.

Keeping the upper arm stationary and alongside, inhale and then exhale while straightening out your forearms with your palms facing each other in a controlled motion. Return your forearms to the bent position in a controlled effort. Three sets of eight.

Triceps Stretch

Shoulders

Military Press

Stand with elbows bent alongside chest, palms facing forward at shoulder height. In a smooth, controlled motion, extend arms straight up until your hands are as far up as they'll go, directly above the shoulders. Slowly bring your hands back down until arms are bent at your sides again and your palms are once again at shoulder height. Three sets of eight.

Shoulder Stretch

Cool-Down Stretch

Biceps Stretch
Triceps Stretch
Shoulder Stretch
Chest Stretch
Upper-Back Stretch

Day 7

The seventh day of each week is the Supa Rest Day. No exercise can be performed without a rest period between sets or individual moves, and no exercise program is complete without prescribed rest. Remember that rest days are as active and integral a part of your workout as breaking a sweat—not a pass to relapse into unconscious eating.

THE WORD

Fitness master Mark Jenkins, author of *The Jump Off* and co-owner with his wife, Natasha, of International Fitness, counts Sean Combs, Mary J Blige, LL Cool J, Beyonce Knowles, Busta Rhymes, and a galaxy of other stars among his clients.

"I get tagged as a celebrity trainer or a hip-hop trainer," Mark told me recently, "but in truth, I train Fortune 500 CEOs and all kinds of people. The more people you educate, and the more people you empower through fitness, the more they're likely to take that empowerment into other areas of their life—lose weight, get your business and life in place, and all of that. Most of the people I'm training now are fairly successful already. You can't always tell them that being more in shape will make them more successful, but what you can tell them is that they can prolong their success and pass along and instill their knowledge. It's a socioeconomic thing. People who are wealthy, who have money, they want me to teach them and their kids about health and fitness so that they pass along that lineage and remain the dominant force on the planet. There's nothing wrong with that. That's what every father's supposed to do. I'm not knocking that.

"It's just that once it gets below a certain economic level, that's not deemed acceptable," Brother Jenkins said. "Those are the kids who are living on prescription drugs, junk food, ramen noodles with no fiber, soda—those are the people who are being exploited. That's how it is in a capitalist society. Somebody has to be at the bottom."

Mark Jenkins is clear about expectations. "I tell my clients that looking good is a small side effect of what they're actually going to get out of living the fitness lifestyle and being healthy and being conscious of what they eat," he told me. "That's just a small part of it. Working at their maximum, 100 percent, is more like a business investment than a matter of 'Oh, I want to be cut, I want to be ripped.' That's a finite, physical, very superficial point that everyone can relate to. 'You can pay me to help you lose that gut,' I'll say, but then you'll need to build off of that to develop as a person. Living healthy will make them better people, better vessels to absorb blessings, better parents, better fathers. It's going to enhance anything they're trying to do and give them more time to accomplish it."

THE LOVE

"Thou shalt love thy neighbor as thyself."
—Matthew 19:19

It's a nice thought. Been hearing it all your life, right? Too bad our society is totally out of step with its sentiments. Everybody these days is programmed to be extroverted, to think and move and operate and love outside themselves. Family first, right? Not if you haven't performed due diligence on your own sweet self. It's easy to fall into the trap of making time for others but not any for yourself. For people living a toxic lifestyle, family and relationship commitments—even making love—become an obligation or burden based on sacrifice—sacrificing time, attention, and health.

Self-Love and Appreciation

In a community full of sick, tired, pissed-off people who hate what they see in the mirror, the "love thy neighbor" part is hard enough. But for that person in the mirror, it's the act of loving herself or himself that is the nearly insurmountable challenge. Your lover doesn't appreciate you? Your friends don't get you? Your family treats you like a doormat? It's because you don't love yourself. You don't appreciate being you—why should they? Having no love for or appreciation of yourself while hungering for the approval of others is as out of balance and as potentially toxic as a diet of white sugar and bacon. We lead by example in this life. If you set an example by demonstrating self-love and appreciation, the people around you whose approval you crave will either get the message, follow your example, and love you as well, or they will fall by the wayside.

Restating that biblical commandment for the new American century might work better as a flow chart that looks like this:

Love yourself generously, appreciatively, and unconditionally.

↓

Offer your neighbor the same unconditionally generous spirit with which you love yourself.

↓

Go back to rule one.

Each one of the six principles calls back and looks forward to the others. Wellness starts with Will and Desire, but it takes root in Self-Love and Appreciation. Put will and desire to use and catalog the things you appreciate about yourself. Make a list. Open your notebook and write down five things you love about yourself, five things you genuinely appreciate about you. If you're too blocked to make that leap, write down five incidents or memories when you were happiest to be you. Detail where those moments took place, and how they made you feel. I'm not asking you to write a screenplay or your life story. You don't even have to keep what you've written. Simply thinking clearly enough to commit those things to paper (sorry, no computer documents, texting, or e-mail allowed—pen, ink, and paper establish a stronger bond) will make you more conscious and strong.

The goal here is to move inside so that you feel good about working to better the world outside. Each and every person alive on earth is touched by limitless spiritual power and possibility. We all know and sense that. Change is here and we all need to be part of it. But feeling sick and tired all the time divorces our mind and spirit from the messed-up physical reality we're trapped in. People are just not feeling good. And when they don't feel good, they don't want to do good, and don't in turn want anyone else to do good. We feel bad and withdraw into states of fear and self-hatred and negative judgment. We hate on each other and want each other to fail because we feel like we're failing. When you're as sick and tired as Americans are, every relationship becomes dysfunctional—something that needs fixing.

The disconnected relationships we have with our bodies become the template for disconnected relationships with our heritage, our families, our work, our future, and the unified, free-flowing movement toward a positive future. That gap-making dysfunction is the model for our shattered communities, laws and regulations that don't make sense to us at home, and policies that don't make sense to the rest of the world. In order to become a working part of your family, community, and the world beyond, you need to relight the pilot light of life within you that ill health and bad dietary habits have nearly blown out. You're looking to turn up the flame and get your glow on. As you do the work and start to get healthy, that glow is what family and friends are going to see. That inner glow is what brings admiration and appreciation from those around you. But you've got to light it and stoke it and warm yourself in it before anyone else will.

THE WORD

Benjamin Chavis, D.Min.—"Dr. Ben"—is the living embodiment of a half century of struggle for African American civil rights. At twelve, he successfully fought to integrate his segregated local public library in the deep South. During the sixties as a youth co-coordinator for the Southern Christian Leadership Conference, Dr. Ben marched alongside Reverend Dr. Martin Luther King and campaigned for Robert Kennedy. Dr. Ben spent most of the seventies in maximum-security lockdown as an American political prisoner, in the words of Amnesty International—one of the wrongfully imprisoned "Wilmington 10"—before he was finally paroled and exonerated.

His groundbreaking 1981 study on pollution in African American neighborhoods, "Toxic Waste and Race in the United States of America," put the term "environmental racism" into play. Dr. Ben was made the youngest head of the NAACP in its history in 1993. His pioneering work with Russell Simmons and the Hip-Hop Summit Action Network continues to this day.

Throughout more than fifty years of work within the movement, Dr. Ben has remained mindful of the necessity for a conscious and informed approach to eating and lifestyle.

"The connection between one's physical health and one's spiritual health started at a very early age for me," Dr. Ben said. "It's what I would call movement health. You can't change the world if you're not paying attention to your own community, you can't change the world if you're not paying attention to your own body, and you can't change the world if you're not paying attention to your own consciousness. Having a healthy consciousness versus an unhealthy consciousness is just as important as having a healthy body versus an unhealthy body. You have to be able to see life as a journey and make sure that you are doing things in your life that strengthen your health, strengthen your consciousness, and strengthen your perceptions of reality.

"I did everything I could in prison to get out of that prison cell," Dr. Ben explained. "I taught GED classes and taught inmates how to get their high school diplomas. I taught a yoga class in prison. Can you believe that? I convinced the guards to allow me to teach yoga. When they saw the people just sitting there in meditation, the guards were laughing. They thought we were trying to meditate ourselves out of prison."

Working with the Southern Leadership Christian Conference to organize and mobilize citizens on behalf of desegregation was a movement-health workout all its own. "Marching is therapeutic," Dr. Ben said. "When you lift your feet and take steps on behalf of others, that in itself is therapeutic."

Now, through his work with the Hip-Hop Summit Action Network, an organization he founded with Russell Simmons in 2000, Dr. Ben is taking movement consciousness and movement health to a global level. "There's an evolutionary relationship between civil rights and hip-hop. Hip-hop grew out of the civil rights movement. And both the hip-hop movement and the civil rights movement have higher aspirations. Sometimes people misunderstand hip-hop and say that it's overly materialistic. 'Bling-bling' is not so much about materialism as it is about wanting something better and how you define what is better. People want a better quality of life; people want to see more peace in the world, less violence and less self-destruction. So if you look at the lyrics of the early hip-hop and even the lyrics today, very often you will find lyrical content that speaks of living well . . . And part of living well is having good health."

three

Week Two—The Vegetarian

Week Two moves us deeper into vegan territory. For the next seven days, you'll have a fresh vegetable intake that balances about 50–75 percent live and uncooked fruit, vegetables, and grains with between 25 and 50 percent that have been steamed or lightly sautéed to retain as much of their living nutrient enzymes, cleansing water, and oxygen as possible.

In Week Two, we are going to swear off:

- ✗ Chicken
- ✗ Fish
- ✗ Dairy: milk, butter, eggs, etc.

THE TRUTH

Commercially raised chickens and eggs are a toxic-additive smorgasbord. Even free-range chicken is unfit for human consumption, due to the absence of fiber in its flesh. The world's fish supplies are dwindling and our oceans and lakes are growing more and more contaminated. Reduce fish intake to zero for the remaining four weeks of the Supa Power Plan and eliminate another major source of toxins in your diet.

Dairy has three big strikes against it.

1. It's High-additive.

* Dairy cows are injected with a pharmacopeia of drugs and antibiotics.
* The pesticides and chemicals in cows' grain feeds are transferred to humans who drink cow's milk.
* The infections and other organic contaminants dairy cows are exposed to in factory farms are also present in their milk and therefore in the people who drink it.

2. It's Low-nutrient.

* Though cow's milk starts out at a fairly sympathetic pH for humans, once it's pasteurized and homogenized, it's too acid to sustain homeostasis.
* Pasteurization kills much of the vitamins and enzyme nutrition that cow's milk is supposed to pass on to calves. A calf raised on pasteurized milk will, in fact, starve.

3. It's Genuinely Bad for You.

* The nutrient recipe in cow's milk is meant for a developing animal with a small brain, big skeleton, and four-part stomach, not you—a grown animal with a big brain, small skeleton, and one-part stomach. It makes even less sense to give cow's milk to human kids—they need human nutrition, not a bovine developmental road map.
* Cow's milk stimulates the production of mucus and makes asthma and allergy symptoms worse, thanks to the milk protein casein—a main ingredient in Elmer's Glue and some plastics.
* A large portion of the population can't digest lactose, a sugar found in milk.

* Pasteurization eliminates phosphatase, an enzyme in milk that enhances calcium absorption. Pasteurized milk actually makes it *harder* to get enough calcium for your teeth and bones.

* Homogenizing milk releases xanthine oxidase—a deadly enzyme that leads directly to hardened arteries, high blood pressure, and cardiovascular diseases like stroke and heart attack.

THE WORD

As the co-originator of the "Philly Soul" sound, Kenny Gamble's music career stretches back decades. But after writing and producing smash-hit records like "Love Train," "Cowboys to Girls," and "If You Don't Know Me By Now," Kenny has become active in humanitarian causes aimed at improving America's health.

"My wife has a program called 'The Wellness of You,'" Kenny says. "From that you learn that prevention is more important than what you do *after* you get sick. Your body is your transportation. You're not going anywhere without it. The better shape it's in, the better quality of life you're going to have. It all revolves around your intake. What you eat and drink is probably the most important aspect of everything that you do. The main thing is to eat fruits and vegetables. That's the number one thing—to get the kind of nutrition your body needs to function. It's one thing to know about it," Kenny says, "but it's another to apply it. We've been applying that kind of lifestyle the past twenty-five years."

THE TRUTH

"Where am I going to get my protein?"

In our culture, we almost exclusively associate protein foods with things such as building muscles and strong fingernails. But that's disrespectful to all the other proteins we ingest. Component amino acids in protein form enzymes, hormones, and cells from the insulin that regulates blood sugar and the T cells that are the foot soldiers of the immune system, along with enough other functions to fill three books. There is much, much more to protein than just muscle growth.

Reality check—the most strenuous bodybuilding we do in our lives takes place as we grow up out of infancy. Human mother's milk, the ultimate custom body-building fuel, allots only about 5 percent of its total calories to protein. If you extrapolate that to an adult of average height and weight, that's a little less than 40 grams a day. The notion that you need upward of sixty to a hundred grams of protein a day—the amount of protein that the meat and dairy industries and the commercially influenced USDA recommend—makes a lot of sense if you happen to work in those meat industries! But you don't need it. And meat and milk do indeed contain lots or protein, along with lots of toxins.

Anything more than 40 or 50 grams of protein a day is actually hard for the liver and kidneys to cope with. Protein isn't an oxygenating food like green vegetables are. When fed excess nitrogen in a high-protein diet, your kidneys and liver create ammonia, which is toxic, slows up your lymphatic system's flow, and rocks the body's pH, too.

The idea of the vegetarian diet's "incomplete protein" is a meat-and-milk-biz scare tactic, too. There are two kinds of amino acids that make up proteins:

*   Essential amino acids—what we need from food
*   Nonessential amino acids—what our bodies synthesize

Yes, beef, chicken, fish, dairy, and other flesh foods have large amounts of both essential and nonessential amino acids in them, along with large amounts of pesticides, growth hormones, antibiotics, and other toxins.

Carnivorous animals have short digestive tracts designed to dump the remnants of a high-protein meat diet. Human beings have a lengthy, meticulous digestion and absorption process designed to assemble protein from multiple vegetable and grain sources, not one-protein-size-fits-all meat and cow's milk. The long, multifaceted human colon also needs a constant intake of fiber in order to function correctly. Meat has no fiber in it. Vegetable protein sources like beans and other legumes are loaded with fiber.

And it goes the other way. While not on the same protein level as he-man sirloin steak, leafy greens and other vegetables and even some fruits are valid protein sources, in addition to being blessed with chlorophyll nutrition, fiber, and water:

✓ Green peas: 8 grams protein per one cup serving
✓ Brussels sprouts: 7 grams/cup
✓ Collard greens: 7 grams/cup
✓ Spinach: 6 grams/cup
✓ Frozen mixed vegetables: 6 grams/cup
✓ Asparagus: 5 grams/cup
✓ Broccoli: 5 grams/cup
✓ Kale: 5 grams/cup
✓ Hulled corn kernels: 5 grams/cup
✓ Bean sprouts: 3 grams/cup
✓ Avocado: 4 grams/cup
✓ Banana: 2 grams/cup
✓ Blackberries: 2 grams/cup

And when you juice leafy greens like spinach and kale, the protein content gets concentrated along with everything else in the juice.

The basic rule of thumb is that muscle-building protein can be had in a vegetarian diet by combining high-protein legumes (peas, beans, lentils, etc.) and/or high-protein nuts and seeds with whole grains in any twenty-four-hour period—rice and beans, for example. True enough, but that doesn't take into account single and complete vegetarian protein sources like:

✓ Tofu: 8–25 grams/cup (the firmer, the higher in protein)
✓ Seitan: 50 grams/cup
✓ TVP: 50 grams/cup dry
✓ Tempeh: 15–25 grams/cup
✓ Triticale grain: 25 grams/cup
✓ Spirulina: 16 grams/cup
✓ Amaranth: 7 grams/cup
✓ Quinoa: 5 grams/cup

The bottom line is that a healthy and varied vegetarian or vegan diet will provide more than enough protein to build muscles and power up. When you factor in that the amino acid protein building blocks found in wheatgrass, chlorella, and spirulina are of much higher quality and more readily absorbable than the protein aminos in animal flesh, and that green vegetable protein sources have so many other nutritional benefits, it's just no contest.

THE WORD

Erykah Badu: "My mom introduced me to so many different things. That's what made me understand that the texture of the meat or the texture of the protein or whatever doesn't matter—it's the seasoning. To me, food is all in the seasoning. Even if it's a piece of cardboard, if the seasoning is good, if it's good for you, then that's what's going down. Now, if I get near a pork chop, I don't get sick or anything; I just choose not to eat it."

THE TRUTH

"What about vitamin B12?"

Vitamin B12, an important vitamin derived from healthy bacteria, is not present in most vegetables in the massive One-A-Day portions that the meat and dairy councils insist that everyone needs. Meat harbors significant amounts of B12 bacteria, true enough. But an out-of-balance acid pH flesh-eating diet actually causes our bodies to lose the ability to extract B12 from flesh foods. Recent studies suggest that the B12 naturally present in our body's own digestive bacteria is actually better utilized by vegetarians and vegans because of the additional fiber found in a nonmeat diet.

There is plenty of B12 in vitamin-fortified soy milk, and it occurs naturally in sea vegetables, quinoa, and in blue-green algae supplements like Supa Mega Greens.

"OK, but what about the heart healthy omega–3 triglycerides my doctor told me take in fish oil?"

There's plenty of triglyceride heart lube in flaxseed and borage-derived vegetarian omega–3 supplements.

THE WORD

Public Enemy's Minister of Information (and holistic health counselor) Professor Griff has been on point about conscious eating for decades.

"First thing I do in the morning is drink water," Griff says. "Shortly after that I have to do dark green leafy substances. I don't care whether I juice it, blend it, or eat it. As long as it's dark green, I'm fine. That's the thing to get the engine started in the morning. Blue-green algae, chlorophyll.

"In the refrigerator right now, I do the vegetables, a-to-z. I keep apple juice and orange juice on hand. Water at room temperature and some cold water. Of course tofu's in there. I do the substitutes—the imitation steaks and the imitation bacon and the imitation sausages and the veggie patties and the chicken patties that are made out of soybeans and that kind of thing. But I balance that out. I don't do that every day. I balance that soy thing out. No processed food. I don't do dairy and I definitely don't do meat. I'm not a Starchitarian, so there's not a lot of starch in my system. I try to balance my meals out."

WHAT'S GOOD?

If you factor in versatility, fresh produce is actually your healthiest *and* cheapest shopping option.

PROS/CONS	CANNED	FROZEN	NONORGANIC FRESH PRODUCE	ORGANIC FRESH PRODUCE
Versatile	No	No	Yes	Yes
Has food additives/salt	Yes	Yes	No	No
Processed/heat treated	Yes	No	No	No
Contains pesticides	Yes	Yes	Yes	No
Plastic contamination	Yes	No	No	No

☹ Canned vegetables are heat treated in a plastic-coated can and almost always are packed with tons of salt.

☺ Frozen veggies lighten up on the salt and retain more nutrition than canned, but usually aren't grown organically.

☺ Fresh produce is versatile—it can be eaten raw, juiced, or cooked.

Organic fresh produce is the top of the food chain. That doesn't mean you can only get it at an expensive retail chain store. Back when I was touring with Erykah Badu, she and I sat down with a writer from a vegetarian magazine to talk about wellness and health.

"What does it take to eat healthy and maintain a good diet and lifestyle?" the writer asked.

"A record contract!" Erykah laughed.

Erykah and I were in Los Angeles at the time, and in L.A., health and nutrition are an obsession. Everybody, and I mean everybody, works out, and stays on point in search of the latest eating and supplement trends. It's a billion-dollar business in California. Warehouse-sized chain stores like Trader Joe's carry every conceivable form of prepackaged food: canned, frozen, wet, dry, organic, vegetarian, carnivore— you name it. And then there are the superstar stores like Whole Foods, where a healthy diet really goes Hollywood. A studio engineer I worked with recently dubbed everybody's favorite boutique supermarket chain "Whole Paycheck," in honor of how empty his pockets are when he's done shopping.

But you don't have to shop at Whole Foods to get fresh or even organic produce. More and more supermarkets are stocking organic produce, and farmer's markets and food co-ops are on the rise. Even if you do choose to go to a superstar like Whole Foods, you don't have to go broke shopping there. It's all about understanding what's in your cipher and arriving knowing what you're there for.

I've got nothing against Whole Foods (or any of the dozen other organic market chains they own like Fresh Fields and Bread & Circus on the East Coast, Food For Thought and Mrs. Gooch's in California, or Fresh & Wild in the UK). They make an effort to supply their customers with wholesome food and useful information. The company finishes near the top of the list of best places to work for in business magazines every year. The first time I went into one of their stores (in L.A., of course) I was dazzled, the same as everyone is the first time, by the light and sound, the high ceilings, all the good things they had for sale, and all the beautiful girls going down the aisles and filling their grocery carts with the best of the best. But Whole Foods is still a business—a supermarket, to be exact, and like all supermarkets they are in the business of selling. That Hollywood dazzle is part of their pitch.

The ground rules on any shopping expedition are as follows:

* At least a third of your budget is for produce—fresh vegetables and fruit.
* Once again—*read the ingredients!* If you can't pronounce it, don't

know what it is, or if it's not what's pictured on the front of the package, don't buy it.

* When it comes to vegetables: organic beats nonorganic, nonorganic beats frozen, frozen beats canned, canned that's been thoroughly rinsed is better than heavily processed food.

* Even boutique chains like Whole Foods have their own generic brands. They also put these house brands on sale, so look for those.

* Visualize the meals you're going to make and look at what you're buying as a means to that end.

* Stay conscious! The sexy lighting and music in superstar stores aren't there just to make it a more pleasant shopping experience; they're there to lull you into unconsciousness. A supermarket is not a video arcade, gambling casino, or art gallery. Get in, get what you need, and then get out.

* Supermarkets are laid out so that in order to get staple items, you have to pass through acres of impulse-buy junk. Stick to the outside of the aisles, and venture in for what you know you want, not to see what they have.

* Opt for dry beans and lentils (bulk where possible) instead of canned.

* Look for whole-grain rice and dry bean bulk options in the international aisle and investigate ethnic grocery stores for potentially inexpensive grain, produce, or bean options.

* Find a farmer's market. If there isn't a full-time market near you, there may be one that sets up once a week or on weekends. Community centers and various advocacy groups often sponsor or host farmer's markets, so ask around or hit the Internet and see if there's one nearby.

* Find out if there's a food co-op option in your area. Food co-ops usually offer reduced prices in exchange for a membership fee or if you agree to work there for a certain amount of hours a month. They're well worth it.

THE PLAN

WEEK 2 MONDAY

Morning Surge
2 tsp. Supa Mega Greens with papaya juice

Supa Breakfast
Whole oat cereal
Grape platter—purple, green, and red grapes

Midday Energizer
Kidney Cleanser Supa Juice (*see page 203 for recipe*)

Supa Lunch
Tofu and brown rice
Steamed string beans
1 apple

Afternoon Stabilizer
Kidney Cleanser Supa Juice (*see page 203 for recipe*)

Power Dinner
Chickpeas, Zucchini, Mushrooms, and Sun-dried Tomatoes over Pasta
(*see page 197 for recipe*)

Supa Snack
Bowl of sliced peaches

Herbal Teatime
Rose hips tea

WEEK 2 TUESDAY

Morning Surge
2 tsp. Supa Mega Greens with pear juice

Supa Breakfast
2 ripe bananas with apple, pear, and pine nuts

Midday Energizer
Liver Cleanser Supa Juice (*see page 203 for recipe*)

Supa Lunch
Sliced avocado on sprouted bread with lettuce and 1 pear

Afternoon Stabilizer
Liver Cleanser Supa Juice (*see page 203 for recipe*)

Power Dinner
Pan-Cooked Broccoli Jump Off (*see page 197 for recipe*)

Supa Snack
Bowl of sliced kiwi

WEEK 2 WEDNESDAY

Morning Surge
2 tsp. Supa Mega Greens with cranberry and apple juice

Supa Breakfast
Peach slices topped with soaked walnuts

Midday Energizer
Blood Builder Supa Juice (*see page 203 for recipe*)

Supa Lunch
Green Lentil Vegiole Soup (*see page 198 for recipe*) with blue corn chips, salad, and red grapes

Afternoon Stabilizer
Blood Builder Supa Juice (*see page 203 for recipe*)

Power Dinner
Steamed tofu and spinach pasta

Supa Snack
Bowl of melon chunks

Herbal Teatime
Peppermint tea

WEEK 2 THURSDAY

Morning Surge
2 tsp. Supa Mega Greens with grapefruit juice

Supa Breakfast
Blueberry muffin
or
Granola with almond milk
A Granny Smith apple

Midday Energizer
Lymphatic Flush Supa Juice (*see page 203 for recipe*)

Supa Lunch
Soy burger on toasted whole-wheat bun with lettuce

Afternoon Stabilizer
Lymphatic Flush Supa Juice (*see page 203 for recipe*)

Power Dinner
Kidney Bean, Okra, and Tomato Stew (*see page 191 for recipe*) with
alfalfa sprouts

Supa Snack
Bowl of pineapple chunks

Herbal Teatime
Red zinger tea

WEEK 2 FRIDAY

Morning Surge
2 tsp. Supa Mega Greens with orange juice

Supa Breakfast
Steamed peaches topped with soaked almonds

Midday Energizer
Respiratory Cleanser Supa Juice (*see page 203 for recipe*)

Supa Lunch
TVP beef with kidney beans

Afternoon Stabilizer
Respiratory Cleanser Supa Juice (*see page 203 for recipe*)

Power Dinner
Sunflower, mungbean, and broccoli sprouts in pita bread

Supa Snack
Bowl of sliced papaya

Herbal Teatime
Alfalfa tea

WEEK 2 SATURDAY

Morning Surge
2 tsp. Supa Mega Greens w/blackberry juice

Supa Breakfast
Peach slices
1 slice of sprouted cinnamon toast
or
Granola and sunflower milk

Midday Energizer
Immune Booster Supa Juice (*see page 204 for recipe*)

Supa Lunch
Soya franks on toasted whole wheat buns, pear sauce

Afternoon Stabilizer
Immune Booster Supa Juice (*see page 204 for recipe*)

Power Dinner
Couscous and spinach
Broccoli salad with sprouts

Supa Snack
Bowl of orange slices

Herbal Teatime
Cinnamon tea

WEEK 2 SUNDAY

Morning Surge
2 tsp. Supa Mega Greens with papaya juice

Supa Breakfast
Whole-wheat pancakes w/berries and raw agave syrup
or
Blueberry oat muffin
½ grapefruit

Midday Energizer
Colon Cleanser Supa Juice (*see page 204 for recipe*)

Supa Lunch
Chef Ali's Home Style Signature BBQ Tofu (*see page 194 for recipe*)

Afternoon Stabilizer
Colon Cleanser Supa Juice (*see page 204 for recipe*)

Power Dinner
"Beef" TVP Stew Beans (*see page 192 for recipe*) and cole slaw

Supa Snack
Bowl of sliced apples

Herbal Teatime
Herbal dandelion tea

THE BODY

Week 2

DAY 1
Warm-Up Stretch
Abdominal Stretch I and II

Hamstring/Glute/Hip Stretch I, II, and III
Lower-Back Stretch

Abs

Basic Crunches (eight reps)
Slow Crunches
Basic Crunches (eight reps)

Lower Back

Back Extensions, up for eight counts, rest for eight counts; repeat three times

Cool-Down Stretch

Abdominal Stretch I and II
Hamstring/Glute/Hip Stretch I, II, and III
Lower-Back Stretch

DAY 2
Warm-Up Stretch

Hamstring/Glute/Hip Stretch I, II, and III

Cardio

Marching Orders
Step Touch
Begin by putting on some kickin' music and step side to side to the beat eight times, widening your stance as you go to increase intensity. After the eighth time, start crossing and uncrossing your arms in front of your chest to the beat eight times as you continue stepping from side to side. Drop your arms down to thigh level and cross them back and forth to warm up your shoulders for eight more beats. Finally, still stepping side to side, bring your arms overhead and back down to thigh level for eight beats to increase the intensity. Repeat series for three minutes.

Legs
Lunges
Alternate Lunges, two sets of eight on each side
Squats, three sets of eight, resting for thirty seconds in between each

Cool-Down Stretch
Lunge Stretch
Hamstring/Glute/Hip Stretch I, II, and III
Lower-Back Stretch

DAY 3
Warm-Up Stretch
Biceps Stretch
Triceps Stretch
Shoulder Stretch
Chest Stretch
Upper-Back Stretch

Arms
Hammer Curls
In regular biceps curl position, turn your hands so that your palms face each other. Perform a curl as if chopping (hand open) or pounding with your fist (hand closed). Three sets of eight.
Biceps Stretch
Triceps Kickbacks, three sets of eight
Triceps Stretch

Abs
Crunches, three sets of eight, up and down for four counts. Do not pull on your head and neck.

Cool-Down Stretch

Abdominal Stretch I and II
Biceps Stretch
Triceps Stretch
Shoulder Stretch
Chest Stretch
Upper-Back Stretch

DAY 4

Warm-Up Stretch

Chest Stretch
Upper-Back Stretch
Lower-Back Stretch
Side Stretch

Standing with feet shoulder-width apart, clasp your hands over your head and interlace your fingers. Holding the overhead position, gently and slightly bow your overhead outstretched arms to the right until you feel a stretch on your left side. Return to start and then gently and slightly bow your arms to the left until you feel a stretch on your right side. Breathe into the stretch.

Chest

Chest Flies

Lie on your back on the floor or a bench with arms extended straight up over your chest, palms facing in. Inhale as you lower your arms out to your sides, keeping arms straight but slightly bent at the elbows. When your arms are an inch or two from the floor, exhale and power them back up to start position as if you were hugging a giant beach ball. Three sets of eight.

Chest Press

Lie on your back on the floor or a bench with your arms by your sides, elbows bent 90 degrees, upper arms nearly at chest level and your palms facing away. Inhale, then slowly exhale as you raise your arms straight up from your chest until they are fully extended, elbows straight but not locked. Your arms should be in line with your chest and not your head or stomach. Inhale and return the arms to starting position. Three sets of eight.

Chest Stretch

Back

Two-Arm Rows

Feet shoulder-width apart, knees bent slightly, and abs tight, lean forward at about a 45-degree angle, keeping your back flat and your head and neck aligned. Hold the arms straight down, elbows slightly bent. Inhale, then slowly exhale and pull your arms up toward your torso, allowing your elbows to bend and your hands to line up (and slightly pass if possible—though DON'T force it) with your sides about midway between waist and chest. Exhale and return to start with a controlled, conscious movement. Two sets of eight.

Back Stretch

Cool-Down Stretch

Chest Stretch
Upper-Back Stretch
Lower-Back Stretch
Shoulder Stretch
Side Stretch

DAY 5
Warm-Up Stretch

Lunge Stretch
Abdominal Stretch I and II
Hamstring/Glute/Hip Stretch I, II, and III
Lower-Back Stretch

Hips/Thighs

Inner Thigh Stretch I

Sit on the floor with the soles of your feet pressed together in front of you. Keeping your abs tight and back straight, inhale and then exhale into the movement as you gently lean forward from the waist until you feel a stretch in your inner thigh. Return to upright and repeat until you feel confident and loose.

Inner Thigh Stretch II

Sit on the floor with your legs spread open in a V. Keeping your abs tight and back straight, inhale and then exhale while gently leaning forward from the waist until you feel a stretch in each of your inner thighs. If you feel confident and want to enhance the stretch, release the stretch a little, inhale deeply, and lean a little further forward as you exhale.

Outer Thighs

Lying Hip Abductors

Lie on one side, top leg on the floor just in front of the bottom leg. Lift the lower leg a few inches off the floor, then lower without letting the leg rest on the ground. Switch sides. Three sets of eight.

Outer Thigh Stretch

Sit on the floor with your legs in front of you. Cross your right foot over the left knee. Bring your left hand across your body to grasp your right outer thigh. Turn your head to look over your right shoulder and, keeping your back straight, inhale and then exhale while gently pulling your right leg in toward you. Switch legs.

Hip Abduction, three sets of eight

Inner Thigh Stretch I and II

Cool-Down Stretch

Lunge Stretch

Abdominal Stretch I and II

Hamstring/Glute/Hip Stretch I, II, and III

Lower-Back Stretch
Inner Thigh Stretch I and II

DAY 6
Stretch

Warm-Up Lunge Stretch
Abdominal Stretch I and II
Hamstring/Glute/Hip Stretch I, II, and III

Abs

Crunches, three sets of eight
Bicycles
Lie on the floor with your hands behind your head. With your lower back on the floor and contracting your abs, lift both knees and shoulder blades off the floor. Do not use your hands to lift your head. Raise your right knee in toward your chest and bring your left elbow to meet your knee, then switch, raising your left knee toward the chest and bringing your right elbow to meet your knee. Three sets of eight reps each, alternating sides.

Straight Leg Glute Extensions

Get on the floor on all fours, then drop your torso down so that you're supporting yourself on your forearms and knees. Contract your abs and keep your back, head, and neck aligned. Inhale and then slowly exhale while straightening out your right leg, keeping it straight and pointing behind you. Breathe normally and lift up the right leg a few inches, feeling the effort in your right butt cheek. Switch legs. Three sets of eight.

Cool-Down Stretch

Lunge Stretch
Abdominal Stretch I and II
Hamstring/Glute/Hip Stretch I, II, and III

DAY 7

Take the day off. You've earned it.

THE WORD

As lead rapper and songwriter for Grandmaster Flash and the Furious Five, Melle Mel changed the face of popular music. Mel and the Furious Five are the only rappers to be inducted into the Rock and Roll Hall of Fame (in 2007). Through public awareness initiatives, Mel—who recently received his personal training certification in California—is trying to change the American attitude about diet and exercise.

"Diet and fitness for me is a lifestyle issue," he says. "It's just something that you do, know what I mean? With most people it's more like vanity. They might want to fit into something they used to fit into like two or three years ago, they try to get into shape to do that, then they've met their goal and it's done. Or it's cosmetic—you want to look a certain way so you do it until you look that way, then you're done. For me, you have a lifetime goal—you want to live a healthy life for as long as possible. It's the same thing that anyone would hear from their doctor after they've abused their body. The doctor will say, 'Well, you have to change your diet, and you have to get some exercise.' The doctor will tell you that every time. Food is simple fuel for your body, that's all it is. When you put the fuel in the car, you must move the car. If you don't move the car consistently and regularly, it's not gonna run right. That's all it is.

"A lot of people get in the gym and they don't eat properly," Mel says. "They wind up just burning themselves out. If you feel yourself getting sluggish and tired, either you're not getting the right amount of rest, or you're not putting the right supplementation in your body. That's the main misconception that people have with diet and fitness. Everybody has a diet. It ain't like you gotta go on a diet, you already are on one, it's just that it's bad. Even on those days I don't work out, I'm planning and preparing for the days when I do work out," Mel says. "I'm eating accordingly and doing everything that will replenish my muscles to get back in the gym. After you work out and even while you're working out, you're preparing yourself to get back in the gym."

THE LOVE

Look at a retail cipher like Whole Foods, or Pathmark (my local chain in Crown Heights). Even check the way a McDonald's, KFC, Burger King, or Pizza Hut is run. There is a reason that fast-food restaurants are so successful. They have clear paths from the doors to the counter. The menus are organized and easy to read. Everybody working there speaks from a script—no small talk or chatter, just "May I help the next customer, please?" That uniform, uncluttered, spic-and-span, no-time-for-small-talk vibe evokes action. I'm in the door, at the counter, and back out the door in nothing flat. There's hardly any difference between walking in and doing the drive-thru. Fast-food companies know the appeal of clean space and a noise-free environment and that's a lesson we can learn from.

Have a look at where you live and work. It doesn't exactly look like the counter at McDonald's, does it? If your home and your workspace are littered with papers, books, CDs, DVDs, clothes, and stuff that you don't use alongside stuff you do, you need to apply yourself to the task of getting that all in order. When a space is cluttered, it's blocked. And when a cipher is blocked, you don't want to be part of it. If your home and work space is in shambles, you're not really present there. Clutter is noise. It's excess weight, and excess weight in the home is just as much a drain of energy as excess weight on the body. That pile of dirty clothes behind the bedroom door is household belly fat. The stack of magazines or newspapers you haven't read is the equivalent of cellulite.

A day or two before my last fast, I went through my home and gathered up something like forty pounds of books and more than 100 pounds of CDs and took them down to the Salvation Army. With all that crap out of my life, I went into my fast with a naturally strong and easy focus I wouldn't have had otherwise. Your energy and attitude carry a positive charge when you make time to clear out the clutter. I'm not saying that you need to create some fake, corporate environment of uniforms, bright colors, and clever packaging. All I'm saying is that action takes place when you pursue a tranquil space. Tranquility doesn't have to mean wind chimes and scented candles if that's not your scene. But in order to be conscious and to hear and believe and act on what you learn, you have to calm down and turn down the noise of clutter.

THE WORD

Public Enemy's Professor Griff: "I'm very particular about the people around me, the environment that I'm eating in . . . and the whole beeper, cell phone, computer thing? I have to be away from that. That stuff bothers me. I had a security guard company and I used to drive by the nightclubs to see if my guys were doing all right. We had a contract with a strip club and I used to see my guys eating in the strip club! I used to ask them, 'How do you do that? How do you eat with *Shake that ass!* and *Bitch, let me see what you got!* and chicks all up in your face and all these different things going on around you? How can you sit there and eat a burger and some fries?' I don't get it, man. I don't get it to save my life."

four

Week Three—The Supa Raw Food Live Detox

The act and process of consuming food is an amazing and elegant synchronized dance of cells and organs harmoniously working together to welcome nutrition and protect us from toxins. Even before food touches our lips, the smell and sight of it already has us deploying saliva to begin digestion once we take a bite and start chewing. The trip from mouth to stomach, from stomach to upper intestine, from upper intestine to colon, and from colon to flush is a carefully orchestrated symphony of processes that extract the energy, nutrition, and water from the food we consume while speeding along the exit for everything else.

On a Toxitarian diet, the food we eat fights those processes every step of the way. When we feed ourselves healthy food prepared in a way that's sympathetic to our body's digestive and metabolic agenda, the benefits can be nothing short of miraculous. Maybe it's the words themselves, maybe it's mind pollution from the processed-food industry. For whatever reason, some people recoil at the mention of the term "raw food." But even a hard-core Toxitarian encounters raw food.

* Salad
* Hummus

* Olive tapenade
* Pesto
* Salsa
* Sun-dried tomatoes
* Carrots
* Fresh-squeezed orange juice

When prepared with noncanned ingredients, all of these things are raw foods. A raw or "live" food is any meal item that has not been heated above 116 degrees (the temperature at which enzyme nutrition begins to break down) or chemically transformed by additives or through smoking or salting. There is a huge spectrum of nutrient energy in fresh vegetables, grains, legumes, and fruit that is destroyed when they are cooked or altered. The advantages of eating raw food are enormous. The living enzymes in live foods are nutritional gold, yet in most mainstream diets, we discard them through cooking. Fueling your body's cells with living enzymes:

✓ Increases energy
✓ Sheds pounds
✓ Clears skin
✓ Boosts liver function
✓ Boosts immune system
✓ Eases mucus production
✓ Smoothes out blood sugar
✓ Fast-tracks digestion

Arguably, there is not a single body function that doesn't benefit from eating nutrient-rich vegetables, fruits, nuts, and grains in their whole, natural, uncooked state.

THE TRUTH

Of all the diet and lifestyle concepts and alternatives out there, eating uncooked food is probably the oldest one in existence. The Greek philosopher Pythagoras is the earliest known advocate of raw food for cleansing and healing. But the modern raw food movement was pioneered in Europe in the 1890s. By the end of the nineteenth century, cooking, smoking, and salting food had been standard operating procedure for a few hundred years. New scientific methods, especially chemical preservatives, moved the Western diet even further away from a natural, raw state. The result was, of course, a new generation of diet-related disease, including epic rates of obesity.

Raw food is all about the active, living enzymes in food that cooking kills. Like juicing, eating raw food gives your body's digestive organs a much-needed respite from dealing with all of the extraneous calories and toxic chemicals in a "normal" diet. Soothing, and fueling with living enzymes and phytochemical nutrition, raw food will take your cleansing and healing to the next level.

I like to apply raw food prescriptively. I find that when I'm at a low-energy ebb or have drifted into Starchitarian diet excess, the purity of raw food eating gives me a big jolt of energy. The discipline of preparing raw food is also a great way to refocus conscious energy toward living and feeling my best.

WHAT'S GOOD?

Though they are excellent and healthy food choices, we will say good-bye to a few vegetarian and vegan staples for the duration of the Supa Raw Food week.

✗ Tofu
✗ Soy milk
✗ Soy sauce

Tofu, soy milk, and soy sauce are all made through cooking. During Week Three, we only want uncooked, Supa Vital foods going into our bodies. If you're having protein anxiety, don't worry—raw food energy and protein come from leafy greens, legumes, and especially the sprouting versions of both ingredients:

✓ Alfalfa
✓ Fenugreek
✓ Broccoli
✓ Mung Bean
✓ Radish
✓ Mustard
✓ Clover

Sprouts are loaded with minerals, vitamins, phytochemicals, protein, and the living enzyme power of raw food. The more exotic sprouting seeds like fenugreek (a legume seed like a lentil) and red clover are unusually tasty and spicy, and will surprise you if you're used to glumly munching alfalfa sprouts and wishing they were French fries. If you can't find them at your local market, fenugreek, radish, and other spicy sprouting seeds are available for cheap on the Internet. The process of taking them from seed to sprout at home is really simple and only takes a few days.

THE WORD

Professor Griff: "You gotta put living food in a living body. If you're going to put dead flesh in a living body, there's going to be a problem. You keep eating these dead foods, your body's going to respond. The system is going to react and shut down. Just like when you cut yourself—that area around the wound turns real hard and turns dark because it's preparing itself to heal. The body will respond."

THE TRUTH

Remember back in middle school science class when they did an experiment where all the kids got cotton swabs and little vials of strong-tasting stuff, and swabbed it on their tongues to map out the location of the specific human taste buds? You get an A if you wrote in your workbook that there are five taste sensations—sweet, sour, salty, bitter, and savory (or *umami*). Experiencing the taste of food as one of the above or a combination of a couple only makes sense if you're eating a narrow range of processed, salt-and-sugar-heavy foods. Processed foods play to the lowest common denominators of taste, emphasizing the primary sensations of sweet, salty, and savory at the expense of the uncountable possible shadings, combinations, and taste experiences that a natural diet in general and a raw food diet in particular provides.

Technically there are only three primary colors. But the world is ablaze with different color combinations. The pioneering American psychologist William James made a strong case for the existence of four primary emotions—fear, joy/happiness, grief/sadness, and anger. Yet life combines these four emotional states and their accompanying behavior into a trillion different moments, each with its own different, distinct feelings and emotional states. Our taste buds need the same space and respect that we give our eyes, ears, sense of touch, and feelings. A period of preparing and eating raw food needs to reflect that sensitivity.

Ironically, while processed food manufacturers continue to recycle the same handful of tastes, nutritionists and scientists are increasingly discovering that the good old-fashioned spice rack rivals the medicine cabinet for preventative health options. Recent studies show some of the most commonly used spices are themselves so loaded with bonus nutritive value as well as flavor that, ounce for ounce, they even beat out vegetables for antioxidant content:

* Cayenne pepper contains phytochemical compounds that help cleanse the liver and boost the immune system.
* Black pepper promotes a healthy balance of stomach acids and aids digestion.
* Cinnamon appears to help stabilize blood sugar and is a potent anti-inflammatory agent.
* Turmeric, the main ingredient in curry, may help fight cancer and joint inflammation.
* Mustard seeds have loads of selenium and magnesium and help protect the stomach.
* Sage has been shown to improve memory function.
* Rosemary helps improve blood flow.
* Nori seaweed, which is a great salt substitute, helps to break down mucus.

THE WORD

"What you do in life has a lot to do with the quality of what you're exposed to," says producer, author, activist, actor, and emcee extraordinaire Stic.man. Whether recording and touring as half of Dead Prez, publishing *Ammo* magazine, or working in inner-city outreach programs, the quality of Stic's life and his family are tied to the fact that Stic, his wife of fifteen years, Afya, and their son, Etwela, are strict vegans. I asked him recently if there was an *ah-hah!* activating moment of inspiration that led him on the path to vegan consciousness.

"I'm still looking for it," Stic said. "I'm still on it. It's a constant thing. There's a real sharp learning curve when it comes to what your body needs and what constitutes real nutrition." For many people, the cost can be just as inhibiting. "Yeah, being able to afford the health food store prices and stuff ain't easy, but people make excuses, too, you know what I mean? Produce is truly the cheapest thing in the supermarket. It's just your taste. If you're trying to get the new Tofutti, that's one thing, but the average fruit and vegetable is affordable. There ain't nothing more expensive than losing your life, you know? I take the approach of a hustler, a person in the street who says I gotta get by on any means. I don't care what I gotta do, who I gotta go through—I'm gonna get what I need to get. That's how I look at the food me and my family needs to have. Whatever I gotta do by any means necessary, we're gonna have healthy living."

For Stic.man, keeping healthy is all about balance. "I've noticed that whenever I feel my strongest, sometime after I get my weakest, and whenever I get weak, I find my strength," he said. "I'm trying to stay more in the middle. Even when I'm feeling strong, I know that weakness is just on the other side, if you don't stay disciplined." Stic's always looking to do better. "It's a challenge. I smoke weed and I know that's not exactly the health recipe right there. Nevertheless, it's a lifestyle I grew up in that's still a part of me. I stopped smoking blunts so I could lessen the tobacco, and I try to keep it regulated, and drink water. Smoking dries the skin out and without the extra water sometimes your skin might break out."

Touring life can also take its toll. "Being on the road, as an artist, you can't always get the best holistic and organic things that you need every day," Stic said. "You know, all your nutrients and stuff. But again, I'm so blessed 'cause I live with a holistic health counselor, so she sends me out on the road with herb packs, and that's what keeps me strong. If I was just on my own, I probably wouldn't be able to represent the health movement as much as I have been, so I give all the credit to her."

WHAT'S GOOD?

In addition to the spices described above, the raw foodist's kitchen should also have the following:

- ✓ Natural hummus
- ✓ Natural tahini
- ✓ Raw nut butters (check the label)
- ✓ Sun-dried tomatoes
- ✓ Natural stone ground mustard
- ✓ Pesto
- ✓ Olives (organic, not canned)
- ✓ Fresh garlic
- ✓ Ginger root
- ✓ Flaxseed oil
- ✓ Sea salt
- ✓ Raw cider vinegar
- ✓ *Nama shoyu* (a raw type of soy sauce)
- ✓ Braggs Liquid Aminos (soy sauce alternative that, like *nama shoyu*, is available at any health food store or online)
- ✓ Agave nectar
- ✓ Stevia
- ✓ Honey

Living raw is great. It comes with tons of pluses, including increased energy, dramatic weight loss, and an enormous boost to your immune system and liver. The potential downside is that it can be pretty time-consuming. Some committed raw foodists use dehydrators and often complex food alchemy to make raw food simulations of familiar cooked foods. The Remedy raw food week is actually full of fast and relatively simple recipes. Full-time raw food eaters also usually take antioxidant supplements to augment the cleansing nutritive properties of a raw food and vegetable diet. On The Remedy's raw food week, your liquid meals and Supa Mega Greens supplements will be plenty.

THE PLAN

WEEK 3 MONDAY

Morning Surge
2 tsp. Supa Mega Greens with apple juice

Supa Breakfast
Melon trilogy—watermelon, cantaloupe, honeydew
Flaxseed with almond butter

Midday Energizer
Kidney Cleanser Supa Juice (*see page 203 for recipe*)

Supa Lunch
Carrot "Tuna" with alfalfa sprouts on salad greens (*see page 200 for recipe*)

Afternoon Stabilizer
Kidney Cleanser Supa Juice (*see page 203 for recipe*)

Power Dinner
Veggie Wrap (*see page 201 for recipe*)

Supa Snack
Bowl of sliced peaches

WEEK 3 TUESDAY

Morning Surge
2 tsp. Supa Mega Greens with pear juice

Supa Breakfast
Citrus fruit platter—orange sections, pineapple slices, tangerine sections

Midday Energizer
Liver Cleaner Supa Juice (*see page 203 for recipe*)

Supa Lunch
Bulgur Wheat (*see page 202 for recipe*) with kale, cauliflower, and Indian fenugreek sprouts on salad greens

Afternoon Stabilizer

Liver Cleanser Supa Juice (*see page 203 for recipe*)

Power Dinner

Quinoa and mungbean sprouts with sunflower seeds ·
Broccoli salad

Supa Snack

Bowl of sliced kiwi

WEEK 3 WEDNESDAY

Morning Surge

2 tsp. Supa Mega Greens with cranberry-apple juice combo

Supa Breakfast

½ grapefruit
Flaxseed with sesame butter

Midday Energizer

Blood Builder Supa Juice (*see page 203 for recipe*)

Supa Lunch

Avocado with couscous (or quinoa) and sprouts over salad greens

Afternoon Stabilizer

Blood Builder Supa Juice (*see page 203 for recipe*)

Power Dinner

Cauliflower Power Dip (*see page 199 for recipe*)
Live Spiced Rice (*see page 199 for recipe*)

Supa Snack

Bowl of melon chunks

WEEK 3 THURSDAY

Morning Surge

2 tsp. Supa Mega Greens with 8–16 oz. grapefruit juice

Supa Breakfast

Apple pear sauce with sunflower seeds and raisins

Midday Energizer

Lymphatic Flush Supa Juice (*see page 203 for recipe*)

Supa Lunch

Sprouted vegetable patties with sunflower seeds on salad greens

Afternoon Stabilizer

Lymphatic Flush Supa Juice (*see page 203 for recipe*)

Power Dinner

Garden Greens (*see page 196 for recipe*)

Supa Snack

Bowl of pineapple chunks

WEEK 3 FRIDAY

Morning Surge

2 tsp. Supa Mega Greens with orange juice

Supa Breakfast

2 sliced mangos
Flaxseed with cashew butter

Midday Energizer

Respiratory Cleanser Supa Juice (*see page 203 for recipe*)

Supa Lunch

Broccoli Hype (*see page 202 for recipe*) with avocado

Afternoon Stabilizer

Respiratory Cleanser Supa Juice (*see page 203 for recipe*)

Power Dinner

Guacamole wrapped in a collard leaf

Supa Snack

Bowl of sliced papaya

WEEK 3 SATURDAY

Morning Surge

2 tsp. of Supa Mega Greens in blackberry juice

Supa Breakfast
Nectarines and peaches with soaked walnut blend

Midday Energizer
Immune Booster Supa Juice (*see page 204 for recipe*)

Supa Lunch
Fennel sprouts and tahini on a bed of greens

Afternoon Stabilizer
Immune Booster Supa Juice (*see page 204 for recipe*)

Power Dinner
Grated beets, young corn, cauliflower, and spinach

Supa Snack
Bowel of sliced oranges

WEEK 3 SUNDAY

Morning Surge
2 tsp. of Supa Mega Greens with papaya juice

Supa Breakfast
2 plums
Hazelnuts and raisins

Midday Energizer
Colon Cleanser Supa Juice (*see page 204 for recipe*)

Supa Lunch
Tabouli (or quinoa) and veggie salad with sesame seeds and tahini

Afternoon Stabilizer
Colon Cleanser Supa Juice (*see page 204 for recipe*)

Power Dinner
Raw okra and radish sprouts on salad greens

Supa Snack
Bowl of sliced apples

THE BODY

Week 3

It's no coincidence that heart rates and dance beats are both measured in BPM—beats per minute. In Week Three, we're going to start cranking up the cardio, so choose your workout music accordingly.

* Most hip-hop and rock 'n' roll ranges between 75 and 100 BPM.
* House, jungle, and drum-and-bass can crank it up to 200 BPM.
* Speed metal can go even faster.

Your heart rate BPM is a good measure of how hard you are working out. Start with your maximum heart rate. To figure out your maximum heart rate, simply subtract your age from 220. If you are 40, for example, your maximum heart rate (220–40) is 180.

For a low to moderate workout, your heart rate should be 60–65 percent of your maximum heart rate. For a high-intensity workout, your heart rate should be 80–85 percent of your maximum heart rate. To figure out the appropriate heart rate, multiply your maximum heart rate by the percentage of intensity you wish to maintain. So if you're still 40, and are reaching for 65% intensity, your target heart rate is 117 (.65×180 =117). Looks like it's house jams for you.

To measure your heart rate, place the index and middle fingers of your left hand on your wrist, about an inch above the base of your hand, in line with the thumb on that hand. When you feel a pulse, gently press down and begin counting for 10 seconds. Multiply this number by 6 to calculate your heart rate. For example, if you have counted 15 pulses in 10 seconds, your heart rate is 90 beats per minute. Got it?

Also this week, we'll begin using optional weights to add difficulty to your workout and definition to your body sculpting. You can buy one-pound barbells just about anywhere, but if money's too tight, an unopened can of soup or beans weighs about a pound, too. You can also use a one-pound bag of rice or dried beans, but be careful, as the bag can rip.

For a medicine ball alternative, I recommend using a plastic gallon jug, just like the one I prefer for the Remedy Cleanse. Completely filled, a gallon jug weighs about 8.5 pounds. You can of course drain it, if that's too heavy at first.

THE WORD

Public Enemy's founder, Chuck D: "I think one of the things that helped us in PE was our regimen of faster songs and movement. It was really simple—you do the song or the song's gonna do you. You know 'Bring The Noise' was a hundred and nine beats per minute? You can't do that just standing there. It was athletic. At that speed and that length, it's like a decathlon. With the fast speeds, you're rapping and you're moving—it ain't like you're standing in one place. So that gave me my workout. Flava [Flav] would run around and I would run with him, and that gave him his workout. The act itself would work us out."

Professor Griff: "I don't mean to be all funny and jovial about it, but sometimes you need to be in order to digest the truth. Shit, I had to keep up with Flava's ass and how bad he is. I had to get my diet right, because that dude stays up all night and sleeps all day. And then on stage it's just ridiculous. A damn two-hour show with a cat like Flava? Oh no, man, you gotta be able to keep up with him, you know what I mean? You gotta be alert man, for real."

Day 1

Warm-Up Stretch
  Abdominal Stretch I and II
  Hamstring/Glute/Hip Stretch I, II, and III

Cardio

Step Touch crossing arms over chest, thighs, and overhead, eight times each. Try to bringing your knees up in front of you as high as they'll go on each step. Repeat series for three minutes.

Arms

Biceps Stretch

Biceps Curls, 1 lb. weight or one 16 oz. can in each hand, three sets of eight

Triceps Stretch

Triceps Press (see page 159) 1 lb. weight or one 16 oz. can in each hand, three sets of eight

Abs

Crunches, three sets of eight.

Back

Lower-Back Extensions, lift for eight counts, rest for eight counts. Repeat three times.

Cool-Down Stretch

Biceps Stretch

Triceps Stretch

Lower-Back Stretch (Standing)

Abdominal Stretch I, II, and III

Day 2

Warm-Up Stretch

Hamstring/Glute/Hip Stretch I, II, and III

Lunge Stretch

Lower-Back Stretch

Legs

Lunges

Lunge with left leg, hold lunge, lower right knee toward (but not all the way to) the floor, eight times. Staying in lunge, lower right knee for two counts and then raise it for two counts, four times. Single lunges, eight times. Repeat with right leg forward.

Squats

Feet shoulder-width apart, single squat eight times. Staying in squat, lower two counts, raise two counts, four times. Stay in squat, tiny pulses, sixteen times. Single squats, eight times.

Glutes

Standing Leg Raises

Face the wall about two feet from it. Place hands on the wall at mid-chest height to balance. Exhale and bring your right leg up behind you as far as it will comfortably go. Keeping the angle, raise your leg up until your right foot is at the height of your lower back. Repeat sixteen times, then switch legs.

Stretch

Lunge Stretch
Hamstring/Glute/Hip Stretch I, II, and III
Outer Thigh Stretch
Inner Thigh Stretch
Abdominal Stretch I and II

Day 3

Stretch

Chest Stretch
Upper-Back Stretch
Lower-Back Stretch

Side Stretch
Abdominal Stretch I and II

Chest

Chest Presses, 1 lb. weight or one 16 oz. can in each hand, three sets of eight
Chest Flies, 1 lb. weight or one 16 oz. can in each hand, three sets of eight
Chest Stretch

Back

Two Arm Rows, 1 lb. weight or one 16 oz. can in each hand, two sets of eight
Upper-Back Stretch
Lower-Back Stretch

Abs

Crunches, eight sets
Bicycle Crunches, alternating eight: four right elbow–left knee, four left elbow–right knee. Repeat above series three times, resting for one minute in between.
Abdominal Stretch I and II
Abdominal Stretch III
After Abdominal Stretch II, gently bring your bent knees to the floor on the right side of your body while keeping your torso square to the ceiling. Swing your arms to the floor together on the left side of your body and look toward your arms, feeling a gentle stretch on through the right side abs (obliques). Gently bring the knees center and reverse to achieve the same stretch on your left obliques.

Cool-Down Stretch

Chest Stretch

Upper-Back Stretch
Lower-Back Stretch
Side Stretch

Day 4

Warm-Up Stretch
Triceps Stretch
Biceps Stretch
Upper-Back Stretch
Shoulder Stretch
Lunge Stretch
Hamstring/Glute/Hip Stretch I, II, and III
Outer Thigh Stretch
Inner Thigh Stretch

Shoulders
Military Press, 1 lb. weight or one 16 oz. can in each hand, three sets of eight
Shoulder Stretch

Cardio
Step Touch, crossing chest, low, and overhead, and lifting knees high, eight times each for three minutes. March in place for one minute, getting knees as high up as you can without losing balance.

Legs
Calf Raises
Stand facing the wall, hands on the wall for balance. Standing upright, raise heels off the ground. Lower the heels but don't touch down. Repeat eight times for three sets total (twenty-four reps). Inhale as you come down, exhale as you go up. To stretch, lean against the wall with one leg behind you, then switch legs.

Cool-Down Stretch

Lunge Stretch
Hamstring/Glute/Hip Stretch I, II, and III
Outer Thigh Stretch
Inner Thigh Stretch

Day 5

Warm-Up Stretch

Hamstring/Glute/Hip Stretch I, II, and III
Abdominal Stretch I, II, and III
Outer Thigh Stretch
Inner Thigh Stretch

Cardio

Step Touch with arms coming overhead eight times. Add alternating hamstring butt kicks—as you plant your left foot, bend the right knee and bring your right foot back and up as if trying to kick your butt with your right heel. Plant the right foot and lift your left foot back as if to kick your butt with your left heel. Alternate eight times each side.

Keep alternating the butt kicks, and put your arms out in front of you at waist height and pull your arms back and forth like in a row exercise, with palms up and elbows bent, in time with the beat, and with butt kicks, eight times. High-knee march in time, eight times. Step Touch with deep breaths in and out, eight times. Repeat series for three minutes.

Standing Hip Abductors

Stand with left hand against a wall for balance. Inhale and exhale while gently lifting the right leg to the side until it is hip height (or as close as you can get it). Do not strain your hip. Let your right leg go down in a controlled motion. Repeat eight times. Switch sides. Three sets of eight.

Legs

Plié Squats

Stand with your feet outside, shoulder-width apart, toes and knees pointing to the corners of the room. Without letting your knees move ahead of your toes (you may have to fine-tune your stance) and keeping your back straight, inhale and then exhale and lower your butt down by contracting your inner thighs. Pause and come back up. Three sets of eight.

Lower-Back Stretch

Medicine Ball Wood Chop

Standing with feet shoulder-width apart, carefully grip the medicine ball (or jug) up over your head. Inhale, and as you exhale come down into a squat while swinging the ball down in a controlled complementary motion until it's hanging between your thighs and your elbows are against your inner things. On the exhale come up out of the squat and slowly lift the ball back to the start position, twelve times.

Abs

Medicine Ball Obliques

Standing with feet shoulder-width apart, hold the ball or jug with both hands, elbows bent, waist height. Keeping your feet stationary, twist your torso and bring the ball to your right, back to center, and left, feeling the pump in your sides and abs. Breathe evenly. Repeat fifteen times.

Bicycles, three sets of eight.

Cool-Down Stretch

Inner Thigh Stretch

Hamstring/Glute/Hip Stretch I, II, and III

Abdominal Stretch I, II, and III

Side Stretch

Day 6

Warm-Up Stretch
Hamstring/Glute/Hip Stretch I, II, and III

Cardio
First Segment, One Minute Each (Medium or High Intensity Optional)
Low Intensity: March in place
Medium Intensity: Jog in place
High Intensity: Jog in place, bringing knees up as far as they'll safely go (no pain or loss of balance)

Second Segment, One Minute Each (Medium or High Intensity Optional)
Low Intensity: Standing hamstring butt kicks
Medium Intensity: Hamstring butt kicks alternating with knee bends
High Intensity: Jog in place, legs behind, kicking your own butt

Third Segment, One Minute Each (Medium or High Intensity Optional)
Low Intensity: Standing alternate knee raises
Medium Intensity: Bring knees up higher, bringing arms over head with each raise
High Intensity: Jog in place, bringing knees way up and pump arms like you're running

Cool-Down Stretch
Hamstring/Glute/Hip Stretch I, II, and III

Day 7

Have a green juice and chill. Spend some time picking out music to work out to in Week Four.

THE LOVE

When you see the word "discipline," what do you picture? A boot-camp drill instructor screaming? A death-row inmate marking time with push-ups? A monk denying himself pleasure of any kind? A dominatrix in leather? In our culture, we've grown so slack and so good at surrendering, taking the short-haul, easy way out of a long-haul life, getting steamrolled by bad habits, that the word "discipline" has come to mean "punishment."

The actual Latin root of "discipline" is *discipulus,* meaning "student." True discipline has nothing to do with pain or punishment. Exerting discipline isn't giving yourself stitches by candlelight or enduring a beating. It's the absolute opposite of self-denial. Discipline is all about learning. It builds and feeds on those *ah-hah!* moments when information becomes active, alive, and applied, and understanding becomes *overstanding.* When you exert discipline you are a disciple—a devoted and avid student of the art and science of living well and energetically, without illness or pain.

Discipline is exercising curiosity—building on what you know and feel and hungering to know and feel more. Discipline is taking the time to ask questions, listen to the answers, and make sure that you're satisfied with what you hear. Discipline is practicing a wellness regime that works for you and challenges you to live the best that you can. It's not a death march; it's not a life sentence—it's your wings over prison walls, your "get out of jail free" card. Discipline is freedom.

With sources of noise gone from your life, you can better listen for the call-to-action, *ah-hah!* moments that living consciously brings on, like bees to flowers. Knowledge is powerful, but the activation and truthful, complete absorption of that knowledge is what really turns on the juice. The stuff we're dealing with needs to go into your mind with the authority of an *ah-hah!* or *Eureka!* revelation moment. It's pretty easy to understand what's making you sick and tired. But in order to cultivate the discipline of putting that info into action, you need to have a moment of overstanding. Understanding is a nodding head, a "yeah, sure, drink water nonstop, more vegetables, less meat, get a juicer, work out, I got it, I got it" level of absorption. C'mon, you know all that stuff already anyway. If merely understanding that could change your life, you'd be out on the dance floor now instead of reading this book.

Overstanding means that the information has struck the *ah-hah!* chord and is active and live inside of you. Overstanding is the third beat—the reestablishment of flow from one good choice to the next. Fueled by the will and desire that's consciously pushed you toward enlightenment, tempered by the self-love and appreciation that makes it worthwhile, you actively overstand what it takes to walk the wellness walk, not just hear the talk. The enemy of depression is action. Positive, flowing progress and a move away from negative, unwilling, self-hating depression begins when you cut the noise, hear and overstand the *ah-hah!* truth, and activate as the disciple of wellness that you are!

THE WORD

Ben Chavis: "Whatever your diet is, be disciplined about it. When you go off of a diet, you're not cheating the diet—you're cheating yourself. There's a myth out there that happiness is the absence of discipline. Some people think engaging in self-discipline is not a joyful thing. But I find it just the opposite."

five

Week Four—Supa Seven-Day Juice Fast

"Cleanliness is next to godliness," right? Fasting—cleansing the body through the controlled, intentional, and temporary abstinence from food intake—has been a cornerstone of human health for as long as there have been humans. Lent, Ramadan, Yom Kippur—nearly every religion equates fasting with spiritual purity. Fasting is advocated or described in the Old and New Testaments (dozens of times), the Koran, the Torah, and Buddhist scriptures. No wonder—the health benefits, the supercharge of energy, and the incredible sensation of awakening and focus that come with fasting are nothing short of a divine revelation.

Regardless of your religious background, fasting for health is the ultimate way to detox. You've experienced how The Remedy Cleanse's potent mix of detoxing, nutrition boost, and flushing improves how you feel and look. Week Four's Supa Seven-Day Juice Fast takes that healthy, high-nutrition cleanse to the next level.

THE TRUTH

On a modern junk-food diet, it's possible to effectively starve on 3,000 empty-additive and toxin-heavy calories a day. With the ravages of that kind of conspicuous consumption showing up more and more as disease, fasting for health is gaining traction, especially in the body-conscious, success-driven world of entertainment. Master Cleanse, açai berry, water fasts—there are literally dozens of types and styles of fasts popping up and as many stated health goals to go with them. You probably know someone who's tried at least one of the fasts going around these days.

The absurd amount of heavy meat meals and simple-carbohydrate starchy foods of sketchy quality that we eat in America makes us perfect candidates for exploring the health benefits of a juice fast. Temporarily refraining from eating solid food gives our organs a vacation from the ravages of poor diet and gives our body's natural cleansing abilities an opportunity to catch up on a backlog of environmental poisons all that bad food has been preventing it from purging. A periodic, carefully structured juice fast helps your cells to rid themselves of toxins, greatly enhances your metabolic system, and turns back the clock on the destruction that years of bad diet causes.

✓ Reduced carbohydrate and calorie intake—empties the liver's carbohydrate stores and puts fat cells to work as food.
✓ Reduced toxin intake—soothes the liver, kidneys, immune, and lymph systems.
✓ Ramped-up phytochemical, enzyme, vitamin, and mineral nutrition—pampers every cell in your body.

Bathing your stomach, colon, liver, kidneys, pancreas, lymphatic system, muscles, lungs, brain, and everything else in naturally highly nutritious and alkaline pH juice and green food supplements shifts your body into one of the most beneficial modes possible. This absence of solid food (but abundance of nutrition) is the climax of the detoxing through diet we've been doing up until now. In the scrupulously maintained alkaline pH environment the fast creates, and without a constant, readily available source of excess glycogen from food, your cells clean house. The fat stored in your liver and in fat cells throughout your body is finally put to good use, as are sick or dead cells that would ordinarily be passed over when conventional solid food nutrition and energy stores are available as fuel. On a juice fast, your internal mechanisms perform their own version of surgery and liposuction by devouring bad and dead cells and consuming excess fat. Your body metabolizes your excess fat stores and damaged cells and dumps the toxins stored along with them. The juice-fast cocktail of soluble fiber and water flushes out that fat and toxicity for good.

As the penultimate week of The Remedy Supa Power Plan, a seven-day juice fast is the masterstroke. Once you've come through the Supa Seven-Day Juice Fast, you will be transformed into a full-on Chlorophyllian with the increased energy and sleeker profile that that entails.

THE WORD

"If you have a life preserver and you can see that someone's drowning, why not throw it to them?" asks Doug Green, owner and operator of Liquiteria in Manhattan's East Village. Since 1996, Brother Doug has been offering a citywide life preserver by dispensing 100-percent organic fresh vegetable juices, healthful, natural holistic elixirs, fruit smoothies, soups, and sandwiches to a revolving door of clients representing both the penthouse-trendy present and the old-school immigrant past of this evolving downtown neighborhood. During my recent visit to Liquiteria, as a couple of Lower East Side old-timers compared notes with Doug out on the sidewalk about what juices to drink to heal skin irritations, at the same time models and tourists rolled up to the counter for shots of fresh wheatgrass and cold-pressed juice blends like the All Green and the Immune Booster.

"My family was the largest cigarette vendor in America," Brother Doug told me, "but my mother was part of the sixties and all the teachings and readings and travel brought her down a path of enlightenment." At the same time that Doug's mom was juicing and supplementing,

"I was going to schools and hospitals and institutions and filling up machines with snacks and gum."

In Liquiteria, Doug has found a totally positive way to combine both his mother's teachings and his family's entrepreneurship. "It wasn't enough for me to live this lifestyle by myself," he says. "I took it a step further and opened a business." But what Doug is selling has nothing to do with hustling. "People need a respite, they need a sanctuary. Whether it's through fresh juices, our soups, fresh tea, herbs, tonics and elixirs, or the flowers and professional education, we offer a total experience.

"What you need to consume are the things your body is made up of, the minerals, the enzymes, the vitamins, the amino acids," he said. "By consuming those things, you're allowing your body to heal itself and cleanse itself and take care of itself and provide its own energy source. The right stuff is out there to be had," Doug says, it's just a matter of knowing where to look and what to ask for. "There's tons of superfoods out there, green foods, green cereal grasses like wheatgrass, different algae from different water sources around the world, whether it's blue green algae or spirulina or chlorella. These are very deep, rich foods that provide people with a lot of nutrients that they could blend into shakes or use separately to provide them with an abundant amount of nutrients, even if they can't get access to vegetables."

Sometimes it takes a familiar face to get that message across. According to Doug, "That's the upside of all this crazy celebrity worship in this country. Russell Simmons, Julia Roberts, Rosie Perez, Natalie Portman, Jon Voight, the Beastie Boys guys, yeah, they've all been customers here," he says, casually ticking off enough names for a whole doctor's office worth of *People* magazine covers. "Man, Q-Tip has been in here since day one." The same wisdom that lures in the marquee names is true talk for everyone. "When people spot someone like Russell Simmons in here, a lightbulb goes off in their heads," Doug says. "They'll spot someone famous or see a picture of Natalie Portman or whoever drinking a Liquiteria juice in the *Post* and hit the brakes and say, 'Hey, let me go in there, try something, and see what they have.' There's no wrong reason for coming here, or for even just deciding to get a juice at a bodega instead of some soda."

WHAT'S GOOD?

For the next seven days, we will switch to 100-percent organic liquid juice meals only:

* Two vegetable juice meals for rejuvenation
* One low-sugar fruit juice meal for continuing detox
* Additional supplementation with Supa Mega Greens
* Water
* Herbal tea

Ramping up to a juice fast from a Toxitarian or Flexitarian diet ordinarily requires a couple of days of preparation. It's initially a shock to the habit-driven parts of your psyche to just turn off the solid food supply and go liquid overnight. But between The Remedy Cleanse, the past three weeks of curtailing toxic foods, and the last seven days on live food, you're perfectly prepared to go on the Supa Power Juice Fast.

The seven-day juice fast goes best if you eliminate:

X Coffee
X Caffeinated tea
X Alcohol

And any other stimulants or depressants that have not been prescribed by a doctor.

Without the caffeine and the usual cycle of blood sugar ups and downs, you may find that in the first few days of the fast, you'll want to sleep longer or take naps. Go ahead. Just understand that when you are awake you need to remain conscious (not obsessed or hung up, just aware) of the fact that you are a disciple on the fast by choice and clear about your goals and reasons for why you have undertaken the fast.

Write down your fast goals at the outset. Be honest. If it's to lose weight or because your significant other is doing it, or you lost a bet, admit it to yourself. Keep track of the emotional and physical hills and valleys along the way. If you keep close tabs on the details of the experience this first time, you'll be even better prepared the next time. I guarantee you that if you follow this fast right to the end of the line, the benefits you experience will match or exceed your goals and make you want to do it again in the future.

THE WORD

"I used to be a nervous eater," says music video, commercial, and feature director Jessy Terrero. "When I was doing *Soul Plane,* the stress of the movie got to me to the point where I was eating everything on set. I usually fluctuate between about 155 and 165 pounds, but when I was doing *Soul Plane* I got to 190 lbs. We were shooting long days and eating big breakfasts, lunches, and dinners, and craft services was bringing stuff every two minutes. It was like four months of just eating, eating, eating everything they brought to set. It got to the point where it really affected me." But the experience of doing a cleansing fast got Jessy more lined up as far as nutrition was concerned. "The first time it was difficult," Jessy says. "But once you get past the third day, you realize that you overeat most of the time. Your body just doesn't need that much food all the time.

"Now I'm back to 160 and everybody on set knows not to bring me stuff," Jessy says. "If they do, my assistant makes sure they know that it has to be healthy. In the cutting room they have those trays of snacks, but now it's almost like having a rider when you're a music artist. When I come into the editing room, there's nothing on the table. They know not to put things out." Regular cleansing fasts continue to keep Jessy on point. "I'll do it for four or five days," he says. "It's not about losing weight—it's about setting my mind back to a place where I realize a smaller portion of food is going to satisfy me."

THE TRUTH

Almost everyone, especially first-time fasters, hits the wall somewhere during Day Three or Four. By Day Three, your body is finishing up the adjustments necessary for it to make the most of what you're feeding it, and lighten up now that you're not feeding it what it doesn't need. Your mind, however, needs to catch up. Approach Day Three of the fast with care, and with an overstanding sense of forgiveness and kindness to yourself. If you give in to the irritability that comes with transitioning into full fast mode and break the fast prematurely, you'll miss out on the tremendous energy and mental clarity that are literally only hours away by Day Three. Think of it as swimming up to the surface from deep below the ocean. Experienced divers know that their next breath is only a few moments away. They float upward at a measured, gradual rate so as not to get sick from rising too quickly through the changing water pressure. That's you on a seven-day juice fast. Slowly rising from Day One through Day Two and into Day Three. By Day Four, most people will have broken the surface and felt the light of the sun inside them and out and breathed the air with renewed gratitude and energy.

A juice fast is a completely safe, temporary regimen. Nevertheless, it's not something you should do if you're pregnant or nursing. Consult with your doctor if you have any anxiety about doing a juice-fast cleanse, and especially if you have Type I or Type II diabetes, hypoglycemia, anemia, a history of behavioral illnesses involving food such as anorexia or bulimia, or are being treated for any autoimmune or digestive illnesses.

Breaking the juice fast:

DAY 8

Vegetable juice breakfast
Clear soup lunch
Fruit juice afternoon surge
Small salad dinner

DAY 9

Small fruit breakfast
    Any fresh vegetable juice combination
Regular lunch. You have broken the fast.

THE TRUTH

The pioneering developer of juicing for health was an English scientist named Dr. Norman Walker. The first subject whom that Dr. Walker treated was himself. At the beginning of the last century, Dr. Walker was experiencing symptoms that were relatively new then but are sadly the norm today. Feeling run-down and tired, plagued by head and body aches and diagnosed with liver toxicity, the doc hit the books. What he decided was to operate from the assumption that the symptoms he was experiencing were being intensified, if not caused outright, by the polluted environment and organ meat–heavy British diet he was consuming. Dr. Walker radically shifted his diet to one almost exclusively of uncooked vegetables and fruit and began improving immediately.

In 1930, a brush with liver disease pushed him one more important step closer to a life centered on preventive health. Realizing that he could reap concentrated benefits for his liver by concentrating the good things in the raw fruit and vegetables he was already eating, Dr. Walker invented a device called the Norwalk Juicer that is still being used today.

The Norwalk and other cold-press juicers (like the ones my man Doug Green uses at Liquiteria) do such a fine job of dividing up vegetables and fruit into juice and everything else that it produces a pulp that's almost bone-dry. And the "liquor" that comes out the other side is out of this world. Rich in antioxidant vitamins and minerals, fresh-pressed vegetable and fruit juices turn familiar ingredients into exotic elixirs full of the stuff your cells need most.

Juicing concentrates phytochemicals to such a powerful degree that performing a juice fast based around deep-colored green, orange, and red vegetables and fruits carries a remarkable potential to rehabilitate and heal abused cells and organs. Though phytochemcial-rich plants and herbs have been successfully used for centuries to treat infections and illnesses, Western science is currently still in the process of identifying and naming the chemical compounds behind these processes.

So far nearly a thousand different phytochemcials have been identified in plant foods. Among the most potent healers of those are carotenoids found in plant pigments. They include:

* Beta carotene: Also known as vitamin A, present in orange fruits and vegetables like carrots and cantaloupe.
* Lutein: A carotenoid that helps preserve vision and is most plentiful in leafy greens (which have plenty of beta carotene, too).
* Lycopene: A potential anticarcinogen in red-hued veggies and fruits like tomatoes, watermelon, red bell peppers, and red and pink grapefruit.
* Bioflavanoids: A potent class of phytochemicals that you get in abundance from juicing.
* Quercetin: Found in papaya, apples, kale, broccoli, onions, garlic, pears, and cherries; there's also a lot of it in green tea and red wine. It's been found to improve allergy symptoms, strengthen the lungs, reduce inflammation in wounds, and slow cancerous tumor growth.
* Anthocyanins: Found in blueberries, cranberries, and strawberries, they slow cellular destruction and aging.

* Resveratrol: Turns up in grapes and grape juice and is a protective agent for the heart and circulatory system.
* Hesperidin: This carotenoid is found in citrus fruit and is also good for the blood and heart.

Dr. Walker not only invented juicing, he's the all-time champion poster boy for its preventative value. By most accounts he was born in 1867, two years after the Civil War. He died in 1985, six years before the first Gulf War. Do the math—when he died (in a car accident) he was 118 years old! Seventy years of eating raw foods and drinking green juice and practicing applied colon health made him hard to kill. If it hadn't been for the crack-up, who knows how much longer he would've kept going?

WHAT'S GOOD?

A lot of juicing advocates recommend using the juice of a slice of apple or tossing in a seedless grape (grape seeds will stop the cheaper centrifugal juicers dead, BTW) when starting out. True, apple's sweetness blunts the edge of bitter veggie juices like chard, spinach, kale, and other leafy greens and broccoli really well. A couple of seedless grapes will also do wonders for the more earthy and potentially bitter greens, beets, parsnips, red radishes, and turnips. But fair warning—though they're nutritionally complementary and similar in vitamin, mineral, fiber, and water content, your body digests the enzymes in fruit very differently than the enzymes in raw juiced vegetables. Taken together, pure fruit and vegetable juice can clash in the stomach and lead to gas and other mild forms of indigestion.

My recommendation? Go easy on the apple, grape, or any other flavoring fruit addition to a pure vegetable juice combo. Try to embrace the veggie taste and phase out the sweetening fruit as soon as soon as you can handle it. Technically you shouldn't be eating fruit within a half hour either way of anything else, but if that's what it takes to get you juicing, then go for it in the beginning.

A better strategy to enjoying juicing and the juice fast is to experiment with using strongly flavored juiceable ingredients:

✓ Fennel: Adds its distinctive savory/sweet licorice flavor. It's also great for digestion and tough on intestinal parasites.

✓ Ginger root is one of the greatest taste sensations on earth, if you ask me. It also has antibacterial properties, revs up bile production in the gallbladder, soothes the stomach, and helps cleanse the blood.

✓ Parsley has a sharp, punctuating taste and helps the kidneys process and absorb potassium. And it freshens your breath.

✓ Garlic, as hopefully everyone knows by now, is so full of health benefits that it ought to get the Nobel Prize. It's loaded with phytochemical antioxidants that destroy free radical body terrorists. Garlic protects and strengthens blood vessels, lowers cholesterol, heightens brain function, and gives cancer cells hell. In juice, it's delicious.

THE PLAN

WEEK 4 MONDAY

Morning Surge
16 oz. warm water with juice of 1 lemon

Supa Breakfast
4 oz. orange and tangerine juice with 2 tsp. Supa Mega Greens formula

Midday Energizer
1–2 oz. fresh pressed wheatgrass or 2 tsp. powdered wheatgrass or Supa Mega Greens in 8–16 oz. water

Supa Lunch
Kidney Cleanser Supa Juice (*see page 203 for recipe*)

Afternoon Stabilizer

½ oz. liquid chlorophyll in 16 oz. water

Power Dinner

Kidney Cleanser Supa Juice (*see page 203 for recipe*)

Supa Snack

Rose hips herbal tea

WEEK 4 TUESDAY

Morning Surge

16 oz. warm water and juice of 1 lime

Supa Breakfast

Alkaline Cleanse Supa Juice—juice 1 kiwi, 1 apple (cored and sliced),
1 pear (cored and sliced), 1 small finger of ginger root.

Kiwi's naturally high potassium and mineral content along with
apple's and pear's double dose of insoluble fiber in the form of pectin
help bring the digestive tract and, with it, the entire body into healthy
pH alignment.

Midday Energizer

1–2 oz. fresh pressed wheatgrass or 2 tsp. powdered wheatgrass or
Supa Mega Greens in 8–16 oz. water

Supa Lunch

Liver Cleanser Supa Juice (*see page 203 for recipe*)

Afternoon Stabilizer

½ oz. liquid chlorophyll in 16 oz. water

Power Dinner

Liver Cleanser Supa Juice (*see page 203 for recipe*)

Supa Snack

Herbal peppermint tea

WEEK 4 WEDNESDAY

Morning Surge

16 oz. warm water with juice of 1 lemon

Supa Breakfast

Blood Rejuvenator Smoothie:
½ cup cranberries
½ cup blueberries
½ cup strawberries
1 ripe banana
Blend together to form a phytochemical powerhouse that assists your kidneys in purging accumulated mineral salts and toxins from the blood.

Midday Energizer

1–2 oz. fresh pressed wheatgrass or 2 tsp. powdered wheatgrass in 8–16 oz. water

Supa Lunch

Blood Builder Supa Juice (*see page 203 for recipe*)

Afternoon Stabilizer

½ oz. liquid chlorophyll in 16 oz. water

Power Dinner

Blood Builder Supa Juice (*see page 203 for recipe*)

Supa Snack

Lemongrass herbal tea

WEEK 4 THURSDAY

Morning Surge

16 oz. warm water with juice of 1 lime

Supa Breakfast

Digestive Balance Smoothie:
2 cups peeled papaya with seeds
1 cup peeled, deseeded mango
1 cup pineapple juice
Juice of 1 lime
Blend together. This smoothie is loaded with digestive enzymes and will help assuage mid-juice-fast cravings.

Midday Energizer

1–2 oz. fresh pressed wheatgrass or 2 tsp. powdered wheatgrass in 8–16 oz. water

Supa Lunch
Lymphatic Flush Supa Juice (*see page 203 for recipe*)

Afternoon Stabilizer
½ oz. liquid chlorophyll in 16 oz. water

Power Dinner
Lymphatic Flush Supa Juice (*see page 203 for recipe*)

Supa Snack
Red Zinger herbal tea

WEEK 4 FRIDAY

Morning Surge
16 oz. warm water and lemon

Supa Breakfast
16 oz. coconut water

Midday Energizer
1–2 oz. fresh pressed wheatgrass or 2 tsp. powdered wheatgrass in 8–16 oz. water

Supa Lunch
Respiratory Cleanser Supa Juice (*see page 203 for recipe*)

Afternoon Stabilizer
½ oz. liquid chlorophyll in 16 oz. water

Power Dinner
Respiratory Cleanser Supa Juice (*see page 203 for recipe*)

Supa Snack
Peppermint Tea

WEEK 4 SATURDAY

Morning Surge
16 oz. warm water with juice of 1 lime

Supa Breakfast
Juice 1 cup diced cantaloupe and 1 cup diced honeydew

Midday Energizer
1–2 oz. fresh pressed wheatgrass or 2 tsp. powdered wheatgrass in 8–16 oz. water

Supa Lunch
Immune Booster Supa Juice (*see page 204 for recipe*)

Afternoon Stabilizer
½ oz. liquid chlorophyll in 16 oz. water

Power Dinner
Immune Booster Supa Juice (*see page 204 for recipe*)

Supa Snack
Herbal cinnamon tea

WEEK 4 SUNDAY

Morning Surge
16 oz. warm water with juice of 1 lemon

Supa Breakfast
Coconut water

Midday Energizer
1–2 oz. fresh pressed wheatgrass or 2 tsp. powdered wheatgrass in 8–16 oz. water

Supa Lunch
Colon Cleanser Supa Juice (*see page 204 for recipe*)

Afternoon Stabilizer
½ oz. liquid chlorophyll in 16 oz. water

Power Dinner
Colon Cleanser Supa Juice (*see page 204 for recipe*)

Supa Snack
Herbal dandelion tea

THE WORD

"It always puts you in a different space when you get a chance to work out," says Harlem's Jim Jones, founding member of the Diplomats who became a hugely successful solo artist and label head. "It makes you feel that much better. I find my business to be real frustrating, so I make sure I work out every day and let all the frustrations go with a clear head before I make any stupid moves.

"Whether I'm in the studio or I'm touring, I'm working out," Jim says. "I always keep it going. There's always something to do. You don't need nothing to work out. I was very athletic when I was younger. I played baseball, football, basketball, soccer, I rode a bicycle, rode skateboards, played black rope, played freeze tag, ran through backyards, jumped off roofs, I did a lot of things. I also ran from the cops as I got older, so, you know, different things kinda kept me in shape like that.

"Working out has gotten more fun to me as I've gotten older," Jim says. "They say it puts more years on your life and we all need to be in control of our physical side because it helps the mental side. It helps you think clearer. It's definitely a part of my day and definitely a part of my life. And it is a natural high, you know? So, to each his own . . ."

THE BODY

Week 4

All of Week Four includes short cardio intervals to keep the heart rate elevated during your whole work-in. Try to stay on top of the transition time between cardio and sculpting segments. March in place while retrieving your weights or when beginning the sculpting stuff, and make sure to keep your head elevated higher than your heart when you bend down to pick up the weights.

DAY 1:

Warm-Up Stretch

Hamstring/Glute/Hip Stretch I, II, and III

Lower-Back Stretch

Lunge Stretch

Lunges

Monster Walks

Alternate lunge while walking across the room, total of twenty-four on each side.

Cardio

First Segment, One Minute Each (Medium or High Intensity Optional)

Low Intensity: March in place

Medium Intensity: Jog in place

High Intensity: Jog in place and bring knees up

Second Segment, One Minute Each (Medium or High Intensity Optional)

Low Intensity: Standing hamstring butt kicks

Medium Intensity: Hamstring curl with a little higher intensity (alternate knee lifts)

High Intensity: Jog in place, alternating standing butt kicks

Third Segment, One Minute Each (Medium or High Intensity Optional)

Low Intensity: Standing alternate knee raises

Medium Intensity: Bring knees up higher, bringing arms overhead with each raise

High Intensity: Jog in place, bringing knees way up and pump arms like you're running

Legs

Squats, three sets of eight

Cool-Down Stretch

Hamstring/Glute/Hip Stretch I, II, and III
Lower-Back Stretch
Lunge Stretch

DAY 2:
Warm-Up Stretch

Chest Stretch
Upper-Back Stretch
Lower-Back Stretch
Abdominal Stretch I, II, and III
After Abdominal Stretch II (see page 131)

Chest/Back

Wall Pushups

Stand with feet close together, facing a wall a little more than arms' length away. Lean into the wall until you can place your arms on the wall at shoulder height. Step up on your toes and inhale as you use your arms to bring your body in to the wall and then exhale as you push away. The farther apart you place your arms, the harder the exercise. Three sets of eight.

Abs

Medicine Ball Obliques, fifteen reps
Basic Crunches, three sets of eight
Long Arm Crunch

Assume the basic crunch start position but extend your arms out above your head, lightly cradling your head and neck between your upper arms. Perform three sets of eight.

Cool-Down Stretch

Chest Stretch

Upper-Back Stretch

Lower-Back Stretch

Shoulder Stretch

Abdominal Stretch I, II, and III

DAY 3:

Warm-Up Stretch

Hamstring/Glute/Hip Stretch I, II, and III

Lower-Back Stretch

Lunge Stretch

Inner Thigh Stretch

Outer Thigh Stretch

Legs

Standing Abduction, three sets, eight reps per side

Cardio

First Segment, Two Minutes Each (Medium or High Intensity Optional)

Low Intensity: March in place

Medium Intensity: Jog in place

High Intensity: Jog in place, bring knees up

Second Segment, Two Minutes Each (Medium or High Intensity Optional)

Low Intensity: Standing butt kick curls

Medium Intensity: Butt kick curl with a little higher intensity (adding knee bends)

High Intensity: Jog in place, add butt kicks

Third Segment, Two Minutes Each (Medium or High Intensity Optional)

Low Intensity: Standing alternate knee raises

Medium Intensity: Bring knees up higher, and bring arms overhead with each knee raise

High Intensity: Jog in place, bringing knees way up, and pump arms like you're running

Legs

Medicine Ball Wood Chop, twelve reps

Plié Squats

Lower for single counts eight times. Lower for two counts, up for two counts, four times. Lower for four counts, up for four counts, two times. Hold down position and pulse thigh and butt muscles four times. Lower for a single count eight times.

Cool-Down Stretch

Hamstring/Glute/Hip Stretch I, II, and III

Lower-Back Stretch

Lunge Stretch

Inner Thigh Stretch

Outer Thigh Stretch

DAY 4:

Warm-Up Stretch

Biceps, Triceps, and Shoulder stretches

Abdominal Stretch I, II, and III

Hamstring/Glute/Hip Stretch I, II, and III

Lower-Back Stretch

Arms

Biceps Hammer Curls, 1 lb. weight or one 16 oz. can in each hand, three sets of eight

Triceps Presses

Standing with feet shoulder-width apart, bring your arms overhead and bend elbows back so that your upper arms remain next to your ears, but your forearms point behind your head. Keeping your upper arms completely still, straighten your elbows as you bring your forearms back up overhead. One set of eight with no weight, two sets of eight with 1 lb. weight or can in each hand.

Shoulders

Upright Rows, 1 lb. weight or one 16 oz. can in each hand, three sets of eight

Abs

Medicine Ball Obliques, twenty reps

Crunches, eight reps. Up for a two-count hold, down for a two-count hold, four times. Up for a four-count hold, down for a four-count hold, four times. Up and hold crunch and pulse ab muscles eight times. Up for four count, down for a four count, four times. Up for a two-count hold, down for a two-count hold, four times.

Basic Crunch, eight times

Cool-Down Stretch

Abdominal Stretch I, II, and III
Biceps Stretch
Triceps Stretch
Shoulder Stretch

DAY 5:

Warm-Up Stretch

Hamstring/Glute/Hip Stretch I, II, and III
Lower-Back Stretch
Lunge Stretch
Inner Thigh Stretch
Outer Thigh Stretch

Cardio

First Segment, Three Minutes Each (Intensity Optional)

Low Intensity: March in place

Medium Intensity: Jog in place

High Intensity: Jog in place bringing knees up

Second Segment, Three Minutes Each (Intensity Optional)

Low Intensity: Standing alternate butt kicks

Medium Intensity: Butt kicks with added knee bends

High Intensity: Jog in place, adding butt kicks

Third Segment, Three Minutes Each (Intensity Optional)

Low Intensity: Standing alternate knee raises

Medium Intensity: Bring knees up higher, bringing arms over head

High Intensity: Jog in place, bringing knees way up and pump arms

Calf Raises

Right Leg Raises, eight times

Raises, up for two, down for two, four times

Raises, up for four, down for four

Hold raises and pulse sixteen times

Raises, up for four, down for four

Raises, up for two, down for two, four times

Raises, eight times

Repeat for left leg

Cardio, One Minute Each (Medium or High Intensity Optional)

Low Intensity: Alternate heel touches

Medium Intensity: Heel digs, higher intensity, cross arms in front of the body

High Intensity: Alternate heels as though you are jumping rope, add jump-rope arms

Cool-Down Stretch

Hamstring/Glute/Hip Stretch I, II, and III
Lower-Back Stretch
Lunge Stretch
Inner Thigh Stretch
Outer Thigh Stretch

DAY 6:

Warm-Up Stretch

Hamstring/Glute/Hip Stretch I, II, and III
Lower-Back Stretch
Lunge Stretch
Inner Thigh Stretch
Outer Thigh Stretch

Legs

Straight Leg Glute Extensions, eight times
Up for two, down for two, four times
Up for four, down for four
Hold up leg and pulse sixteen times
Up for four, down for four
Up for two, down for two, four times
Up and down eight times

Abs

Crunches, three sets of eight
Medicine Ball Obliques, three sets of eight
Bicycles, three sets of eight

Lower-Back Stretch

Lift for eight counts, rest for eight counts. Repeat three times.

Cool-Down Stretch
Lower-Back Stretch (standing)
Hamstring/Glute/Hip Stretch I, II, and III
Outer Thigh Stretch
Inner Thigh Stretch
Abdominal Stretch I, II, and III
Oblique Stretch

DAY 7:
Rest, but rest strong. You have a big week ahead of you.

THE WORD

Mark Jenkins: "You have to have a certain level of self-mastery before you can effect change inside yourself. If you don't learn that on your own, or if someone's not exposing you to that knowledge, you're risking your life. In a society where a lot of people can't afford health care, it's important to be empowered by knowing about what eating certain foods will do to you."

Mark has learned that ignorance and unconsciousness are what leads to using food as a drug. "We're not eating to perform better, or even because the food tastes good," Mark said. "We're having an unhealthy relationship with an inanimate object. You feel sad, you get something to eat; you feel angry, you take a drink. You have to ask yourself, is it healthy, is it what my body needs to prolong my life? Then, Okay. It tastes good? Even better. Otherwise food is self-medication. I've trained everybody from vegans to artists who eat steak every day to Mafia bosses who drink alcohol all day, a whole variety of people. I try to get them all to understand number one, what their relationship is to food and number two, why they eat what they eat and how it makes them feel. I try to get my clients to write down for a week what they ate and the time that they ate it and their emotions when they ate it, to see if they see a pattern. It helps to get a basic understanding, so that they can become conscious of that relationship they have with food. When a person's conscious they'll naturally want to find out what's best for them. The whole thing is getting them conscious, getting them thinking about it. That's the best way to start."

THE LOVE

Human beings have big brains and deep memories, and we've evolved a complex combination of memory-based emotional mechanisms in order to adapt, survive, and thrive on our decades-long trip to maturity. We formed vital emotional attachments to the parents and other caregivers who raised us from childhood into adulthood. But forming emotional attachments based on need is a tough habit to break. So as adults, we can spend our lives getting hung up on just about anything that makes us feel good or safe.

The sensory experience of consuming food is always emotional. It's a two-way street. Emotional experience triggers hunger, and hunger triggers emotion. Psychic traumas that need sorting out and that unconsciously affect our behavior share headspace with the instinctual need to consume. The pain of one and the relief of the other form connections, and we start using food to soothe our feelings or generate pleasurable sensations offering temporary shelter from whatever personal storm is raging inside or outside. At our weakest, we'll use food as a drug to dull the sensation of pain, soothe anxiety, and hide from difficult situations and events by indulging in a simple, one-way, emotionally centered relationship with what we eat.

Faced with a bad scene, we can easily retreat behind a glazed-over, nonparticipating, shut-down state. Once in that state, the rules governing how we behave, what we eat, and why are null and void. That crisis mode in which we have consciously left the building—even though we're still physically present—is where self-medicating eating habits do their worst. We'll eat ourselves into a false sense of balance and calm in response to any number of emotional triggers hard-wired into our psyches. It's those emotional triggers that allow us to lapse into a half-life of sleep-walking mass consumption of toxic junk, to unconsciously and robotically peel the wrapper off a Twinkie rather than consciously peel a banana, or to gulp down a bottle of soda instead of pour and drink a glass of water.

With will and desire driving you, self-love and appreciation keeping you glowing, and an active approach to discipline reminding you to remain engaged and curious and on point for anything worth learning, it's time to plug up the leaks. Through Emotional Healing we acknowledge the stuff that's just habitual, unmotivated conflict. And by acknowledging it, we take steps toward getting rid of it. Since you're a student and a disciple, you'll need to do some homework.

Experienced fasters know that a seven-day juice fast reveals emotional connections to eating like an X-ray. Use this time to list and study the feelings you have and how they change as your resistance to and acceptance of the fast comes and goes. Keep track of how the physical cravings (and the uncanny lack of cravings that takes over after the first few days) make you feel. Your body and mind are always connected. As your cells and organs dump excess toxic baggage, your mind is likely to as well. Write down the memories and emotional sensations that fasting conjures up. Keep track of the dreams you have while indulging in the extra sleep that fasting often requires. Without all that medicating food and stimulation from caffeine, your subconscious mind really takes flight on a fast. I promise you that you will have some crazy dreams over the next seven days. It's all good, though. The physical and psychological benefits of the seven-day juice fast you are about to undertake will make your body strong and your mind grow more than you ever believed possible. The student's discipline will motivate you. Fasting will unify you.

As you continue through your juice fast, write down the things you know you should let go. Not just the foods that play to your addictive weaknesses but do nothing for you physically, but the behavior and the people who embody pointless, unreasonable conflict. Keep a diary or a list of the emotions you experience on your wellness journey. Note how they give and take depending on how and what you eat, when you exercise, how much rest you get, where you go, and who you interact with. In order to avoid getting caught in the quicksand of old trauma and old habits, it's important to know what is behind your need to vanish when confronted by a particular emotional state. You need to do the work of naming and identifying what it is that causes you psychic pain and propels you into a traumatized, checked-out state where will and desire become paralyzed, robotic unconsciousness; self-love and appreciation transforms into self-loathing and obsessing on others; activation regresses to inertia; and discipline gives way to dropping out.

six

Week Five—Maintenance Week—The Capstone to Wellness

Look at the word *holistic*. **It's pronounced "whole-istic," right?** Whole—as in wholesome, as in unity, as in many parts harmoniously making up the one. That's you, that's me, that's that dude on the corner— each of us possessing an inseparable body/mind, a limitless capacity to do good and the divinely granted ability to form a community powered by health and the strength that health generates.

Unity is a series of circles—the intermingling ciphers that we all travel through. It comes from inside of us. We're made out of it. Unity begins when two cells unite, energize each other, share, and grow. That cell unity widens to include a miraculous and sacred bond between consciousness, bodily functions, and organ systems that, when treated right, work together harmoniously. Unifying flow extends outside of us to form families and create communities. Flow and unity is what nations aspire to—a diverse unity in which the one thing we all share is the dignity, the beauty, and the pleasure of being alive and working and playing, teaching and learning, to our best potential.

Rhythm comes in threes. One, two . . . and? Two beats could be anything. It's beat number three that sets the tempo. Rhythm starts at one and flows through two, then, on three, you're heading for the dance floor or carrying that rhythm in your head and your body throughout the day. Life and music are all about flow. We flow forward in the moment, always in the present as we move from our past to our future.

Over the previous Foundation Four weeks of the Supa Power Plan, we've explored a quartet of lifestyle tempos:

* Flexitarian
* Vegetarian
* Raw Food
* Juice Fast

What beat you make out of those four weeklong approaches to preventing illness, losing weight, boosting energy, and revitalizing is up to you. The next beat, and every beat after that, will be set by you.

THE TRUTH

Life unity is all about cycles. Like the countless ciphers with which we interact and connect over the course of our lives, there are dozens of natural cycles that impact how we live, look, and feel.

* The sun's cycle through the day
* The moon's cycle over a month
* The cycle of seasons over a year
* The cycle of aging over the decades

These things, and dozens more cycles involving hormones, cell growth, blood sugar, memory, cleansing, and a myriad of things on the inside, and weather, agriculture, family dynamics, social pressures, and an equally diverse number of factors on the outside, are proof that:

In life, the only constant is change.

Change isn't catastrophe, it's flow—the natural sequential order of things happening over time. How you deal with that constant flow is up to you. By mixing and matching the four lifestyle options we've explored over the last four weeks, you'll be equipped to physically deal with life's natural and challenging flow of change.

THE WORD

Professor Griff: "When the weather changes, your body changes, and you have to adapt your diet. Although I don't call it a 'diet'—I call it living."

Chuck D: "Ain't nobody living to 175 that we know. Life is gonna deal its own deck of cards at you anyway with uncertainties and unsureties that come along. As you get older, you've got to figure your time clock and your food clock. It's like a body itinerary. The best you can be is stable and try and get ahold of it. You gotta turn down a lot of things. You gotta be mentally strong. Make some kind of itinerary for yourself that combines your mental with your physical: what you're gonna eat, when you're gonna eat it. You gotta make your own map."

THE TRUTH

For the final week of my Supa Power Plan, the training wheels for your ongoing lifetime of holistic wellness come off. If there's a single biggest misunderstanding about holistic living, it's that there are only a few narrow eating options available to you. Compare the variety of meals, taste sensations and food experiences you've had over the last twenty-eight days to the numbing regularity of a sleepwalking Toxitarian diet of snack foods and drive-thru visits and you'll see that it's true. Eating consciously opens you up to a level of sensual enjoyment of food and application of knowledge that cannot be had in a Toxitarian diet.

More important—compare how you look and feel now to how you did on the Toxitarian plan. Depending on your weight, you've probably lost between sixteen and twenty-eight pounds in the last four weeks.

✓ Your body has visibly transformed through exercise.

✓ Your eyes, skin, and hair are clear and glowing.

✓ Your digestion is on point and yielding a healthy bowel movement after each meal.

✓ Your energy level is at an all-time high.

✓ You're aware of your own effectiveness and increased confidence and clearheadedness.

What remains in the capstone of wellness is for you to choose where to go next. Look at the notes you've kept over the foundation four weeks. Are there patterns to how you felt physically and emotionally during each of the Seven-Day Supa Power Plan versions? Most people assume that the plan progresses in difficulty from week one to week four, but that's actually rarely the case.

* Which week was easiest?
* Which was hardest?
* Which week tasted the best?
* Which gave you the most energy boost?
* Which week made you feel the most upbeat?
* Which week offered the most allergy and mucus relief?
* Which week encouraged the most weight loss?
* Which week gave you the most restful sleep?
* Which week had the best exercise progress?

The answers to these questions contain the seeds of knowledge for further application of The Remedy and the tools of the Supa Power Program.

The Remedy and the Foundation Four weekly plans can be useful tools for:

* Preventative maintenance
* Treatment of dietary illness/lethargy
* A boost to help meet a physical or emotional challenge
* Maintaining a healthy body weight

SUPA DIET PLAN	CARBS	ENERGY	CLEANSING	MUCUS RELIEF	DIGESTION RELIEF	WEIGHT LOSS
The Remedy	Low	High	High	High	High	High
Flexitarian	High	Medium	Medium	Medium	N/A	N/A
Vegetarian	Medium	Medium	Medium	Medium-High	N/A	N/A
Raw Food	Medium-Low	High	Medium	High	N/A	N/A
Juice Fast	Low	High	High	High	N/A	N/A

But the choice is now yours. Listen to your body, work out, and eat consciously, and where to go next will be clear.

Food transitioning from season to season can be tricky. While it varies depending on the climate you live in, as fall light turns to winter and long days shorten to early dusk, the tendency is to seek out more carbs as shadows lengthen, and lighter fare as spring arrives and summer heats up. Depending on what you've discovered and observed and what your health and wellness goals are, you may wish to go with that flow by eating Flexitarian during winter's dog days, and move toward raw food in high summer. Or you may find that enforcing a light diet or doing a full-on juice fast or four-day Remedy Cleanse in midwinter may be the way to go. There's a lot to be said for starting the New Year detoxed and cleansed and clearheaded for day one of the next 365.

Allergies pose another seasonal issue. If you're sensitive to mold, dust, plant spores, and other seasonal irritants, it's a good idea to go raw or consider a fast or cleanse during the hardest pollen weeks in spring, summer, and fall.

Also, if you're interested in the grounding personal benefits and giving social benefits of confining your fruit and vegetable consumption to locally grown, seasonal produce, it makes sense to commit to raw food and juice-fast eating programs when the stuff you like the most is available and in season where you live.

THE WORD

Stic.man and Afya have raised their son Etwela on the principles of vegan living and holistic health.

"He's seven years old now, and he's always been a vegan. We never hooked him on things like candy and all that bullshit. He's homeschooled with thirteen other young boys and his primary teacher is reinforcing his healthy diet, too," Stic said. "So he don't really have no big issue with the way he eats, you know?"

What about the rest of the world? Do Afya and Stic have to be on point where nonholistic parents, friends, and loved ones are concerned? "Generally people have been respectful because me and my wife are pretty strong-willed people," Stic said. "My moms and my family and the people around us have been influenced by their health issues and by seeing us, and by hearing us over and over and over and over recommending certain changes."

And Etwela? "As far as our son," Stic said, "he don't really want nothing else, you know? He'll eat pizza sometimes, and bread and ice cream and some other different things. He might say, 'I want to eat some of that, I want to drink that kind of juice' or whatever. Believe it or not, we let him try it and he'll get sick. Not anything that would really hurt him, but little things: mucus, that kind of thing. Then we'll say, 'see, that's why we don't need all that bread.' Basically we just give the responsibility to him and we just guide him because at the end of the day, it's your body and you have to experience it. It's at the point now where if he starts feeling under the weather, he'll say 'I just want to start eating all live food.' He's getting a healthy respect for good food and his mom's a chef, so he likes what she makes, anyway. He and I help her to make the food and so he's become aware of how you create something to satisfy yourself."

THE TRUTH

If you overindulge in alcohol, a meal of raw food (with plenty of raw or juiced cabbage—it works wonders on a hangover) or a liquid juice meal is a great way to get back on track.

If you indulge in Toxitarian extreme eating, a four-day Remedy Cleanse or juice fast is the quickest way to detox, cleanse the colon, and begin the journey back to homeostasis.

For jet-lag and other body clock issues, like changing work schedules, the arrival of a newborn in your home, or bouts of sleeplessness, I recommend doing a juice-fast day while in transit (the flight or day of the schedule change) bracketed by a high-protein Flexitarian or vegetarian day, with meals served as close as they can be to the time zone you're traveling to on the day before and on the day after.

Head colds and respiratory miseries respond best to raw food and juicing. The trick is to let your body's natural healing do its thing. In order for that to happen, you need to give it as little else to work on as possible. Steer clear of Flexitarian days and meals when you have a cold or the flu.

The Foundation Four's weekly meal plans can also be broken down into individual meals. You can do a single meal juice fast before or after any meal. A raw food meal or single juice fast meal and supplementation at the end of the day sets you up for a peaceful mini-cleanse overnight. It's all about what you're trying to make out of your day and do to help maximize your lifelong journey to wellness.

THE WORD

As a Grammy-winning producer, songwriter, and musician, Rodney Jerkins has shepherded the careers of Brandy, Beyonce, and LaShawn Daniels, to name but a few.

"I definitely feel like America overall is getting more health-conscious and wanting to change for the better and do right," Rodney said recently. "In the music industry, you don't have a whole lot of choice. The record companies aren't going to invest money in an artist unless they're healthy enough to sell the product," Rodney says. "It's just like the sports arena or any other arena—you want to look good to sell the product that needs to be sold."

That pressure goes both ways. "Me, as a producer, I'm more behind the scenes," Rodney says. "But I think people believe in you a little bit more when you're in shape. When you're in shape, you can go so much further in life and in other avenues because people want something good to look at. When people see that you're serious about your health, it makes other people want to get right."

Rodney's motivations for seeking an ongoing healthy lifestyle are a little more close to home, however. "I got a little son who's four-and-a-half months and I want to be right for him, you know what I mean? I just think about a lot of times I would get on my father about his diabetes and high blood pressure and things like that and I don't want my son to get on me about it. I want to be there as much as I can. If he wants to play basketball I want to be able to be the coach on his team and not worry about struggling to be that, you know what I mean? It's a lot but it's all good."

THE BODY

Week 5

Week Five alternates sculpt days with cardio/sculpt interval days for variety.

DAY 1:

Warm-Up Stretch

Biceps, Triceps, and Shoulder Stretches
Hamstring/Glute/Hip Stretch I, II, and III
Lower-Back Stretch

Cardio First Segment, Three Minutes Each (Medium or High Intensity Optional)

Low Intensity: March in place
Medium Intensity: Jog in place
High Intensity: Jog in place, bring knees up

Arms

Biceps Curls, 1 lb. weights or one 16 oz. can in each hand, three sets of eight

Cardio Second Segment, Three Minutes Each (Medium or High Intensity Optional)

Low Intensity: Standing hamstring curls
Medium Intensity: Hamstring curl with a little higher intensity (adding knee bends)
High Intensity: Jog in place, legs behind, kicking your own butt

Arms

Hammer Curls, three sets of eight, 1 lb. weight or 16 oz. can in each hand
Biceps Stretch

Cardio Third Segment, Three Minutes Each (Intensity Optional)

Low Intensity: Standing alternate knee raises

Medium Intensity: Bring knees up higher, bring arms overhead, then past the knees

High Intensity: Jog in place bringing knees way up, pumping arms as if you're running

Arms

Triceps Kickbacks, three sets of eight, 1 lb. weight or one 16 oz. can in each hand

Cardio Fourth Segment, Three Minutes Each (Intensity Optional)

Low Intensity: Alternate heel touches

Medium Intensity: Heel digs, higher intensity; cross arms in front of the body

High Intensity: Alternate heels as though you are jumping rope, add jump-rope arms

Arms

Triceps Presses, three sets of eight, 1 lb. weight or a 16 oz. can in each hand

Triceps Stretch

Cool-Down Stretch

Abdominal Stretch I, II, and III

Biceps, Triceps, Shoulder Stretch

Hamstring/Glute/Hip Stretch I, II, and III

Lower-Back Stretch

DAY 2:

Warm-Up Stretch

Chest Stretch

Back Stretch

Side Stretch

Chest/Back

Wall Pushups, two sets of eight, resting for thirty seconds between sets

or

Modified Knee Pushups

From a kneeling position, drop down so that you're supporting yourself with your hands on the floor directly below your shoulders, your arms straight (elbows not locked), and your knees bent. With abs tight and back, head, and neck aligned, inhale and slowly bend the elbows, coming down toward the floor as far as you are able to. Exhale and slowly straighten the arms and push up. Two sets of eight, resting for thirty seconds between sets.

or

Standard Pushups

This is the same as a knee pushup, except your legs are outstretched and you split your weight between hands on floor and the toes and balls of your feet. Remember to keep your back straight. Two sets of eight, resting for thirty seconds between sets.

Stretch

Chest Stretch
Back Stretch
Shoulder Stretch

Abs Set 1: Crunches

Crunches, eight times
Crunches, up for two, down for two, four times each
Crunches, up for four, down for four
Hold crunch and pulse sixteen times
Crunches, up for four, down for four
Crunches, up for two, down for two, four times each
Crunches, eight times
Ab Stretch

Abs Set 2: Bicyle Crunches Right Side
Same series as Abs Set 1
Ab Stretch

Abs Set 3: Bicycle Crunches Left Side
Same series as Abs Set 1
Ab Stretch

Cool-Down Stretch
Chest Stretch
Back Stretch
Side Stretch
Lower-Back Stretch (Standing)
Upper-Back Stretch
Abdominal Stretch I, II, and III

DAY 3:
Warm-Up Stretch
Hamstring/Glute/Hip Stretch I, II, and III
Lower-Back Stretch
Lunge Stretch
Inner Thigh Stretch
Outer Thigh Stretch

Cardio First Segment, Three Minutes Each (Intensity Optional)
Low Intensity: March in place
Medium Intensity: Jog in place
High Intensity: Jog in place, bring knees up

Lunges
Lunge with left leg, hold lunge, lower right knee toward but not to floor, eight times
Staying in lunge, lower two counts, raise two counts, four times

Stay in lunge, tiny pulses, sixteen times

Single lunges, eight times

Cardio Second Segment, Three Minutes Each (Intensity Optional)

Low Intensity: Standing butt kicks

Medium Intensity: butt kicks with added knee bends

High Intensity: Jog in place with butt kicks

Lunges

Lunge with right leg, hold lunge, lower left knee toward but not to floor, eight times

Staying in lunge, lower two counts, raise two counts, four times

Stay in lunge, tiny pulses, sixteen times

Single lunges, eight times

Cardio Third Segment, Three Minutes Each (Medium or High Intensity Optional)

Low Intensity: Standing alternate knee raises

Medium Intensity: Bring knees up higher, raise your arms overhead

High Intensity: Jog in place, bringing your knees way up, pumping your arms as if you're running

Squats

Feet shoulder-width apart, single squats, eight times

Staying in squat, lower two counts, raise two counts, four times

Stay in squat, tiny pulses, sixteen times

Single squats, eight times

Cardio Fourth Segment, Three Minutes Each (Intensity Optional)

Low Intensity: Alternate heel touches

Medium Intensity: Heel digs, higher intensity, crossing arms in front of the body

High Intensity: Jump rope or alternating heel hops and swinging your forearms as though you are jumping rope

Squats

Legs together, single squat, eight times

Staying in squat, lower two counts, raise two counts, four times

Stay in squat, tiny pulses, sixteen times

Single squats, eight times

Cool-Down Stretch

Hamstring/Glute/Hip Stretch I, II, and III

Lower-Back Stretch

Lunge Stretch

Inner Thigh Stretch

Outer Thigh Stretch

DAY 4:

Warm-Up Stretch

Hamstring/Glute/Hip Stretch I, II, and III

Cardio

Step Touch with arms crossing at chest height, eight times

Alternate hamstring curls with two-armed rows, eight times

March with knees high, eight times

Step Touch with deep breaths in and out, eight times

Repeat series for three minutes

Legs/Glutes

Calf Raises, both legs, eight times

Left foot behind right, eight raises on right, trying not to touch heel down between each

Raises, both legs, eight times

Right foot behind left, eight raises on left, trying not to touch heel down between each

Raises, both legs, eight times

Calf Stretch
Straight Leg Glute Extensions, three sets of eight

Abs
Medicine Ball Obliques, twenty reps
Bicycles, three sets of eight

Lower Back
Lower-Back Extensions, gently lift torso and legs, hold for eight counts, rest for eight counts, repeat three times

Cool-Down Stretch
Hamstring/Glute/Hip Stretch I, II, and III
Upper-Back Stretch
Lower-Back Stretch
Abdominal Stretch I, II, and III

DAY 5:
Warm-Up Stretch
Chest Stretch
Back Stretch
Side Stretch
Hamstring/Glute/Hip Stretch I, II, and III

Cardio First Segment, Three Minutes Each (Intensity Optional)
Low Intensity: March in place
Medium Intensity: Jog in place
High Intensity: Jog in place, bringing knees up

Shoulders Set 1
Military Presses, 1 lb. weight or one 16 oz. can in each hand, three sets of eight

Cardio Second Segment, Three Minutes Each (Intensity Optional)
Low Intensity: Standing hamstring butt kicks
Medium Intensity: Hamstring butt kicks with a little higher intensity (knees up high in front)
High Intensity: Jog in place, adding butt kicks

Shoulders Set 2
Upright Rows, 1 lb. weight or one 16 oz. can in each hand, three sets of eight

Cardio Third Segment, Three Minutes Each (Intensity Optional)
Low Intensity: Standing alternate knee raises
Medium Intensity: Bring arms up overhead and kick your knees up higher
High Intensity: Jog in place, bringing knees way up, pumping arms as if you're running

Chest/Back Set 1
Wall Pushups, three sets of eight, try moving the arms farther apart for each set

Cardio Fourth Segment, Three Minutes Each (Intensity Optional)
Low Intensity: Alternate heel touches
Medium Intensity: Heel digs, higher intensity, crossing arms in front of the body
High Intensity: Jump rope or alternating heel hops and swinging your forearms as though you are jumping rope

Chest/Back Set 2
Wall Pushups, two sets of eight, two counts to and away from the wall

Cool-Down Stretch
   Chest Stretch
   Back Stretch

Side Stretch

Hamstring/Glute/Hip Stretch I, II, and III

DAY 6:

Warm-Up Stretch

Lunge Stretch

Hamstring/Glute/Hip Stretch I, II, and III

Outer Thigh Stretch

Inner Thigh Stretch

Outer Thighs

Hip Abduction, eight times

Hip Abduction, up for two, down for two, four times

Hip Abduction, up for four, down for four

Hold and pulse sixteen times

Hip Abduction, eight times

Hip/Glute Stretch

Repeat on other leg

Inner Thighs

Hip Abduction, eight times

Hip Abduction, up for two, down for two, four times

Hold and pulse, eight times

Hip Abduction, eight times

Abs

Medicine Ball Obliques

Crunches, three sets of eight

Bicycles, three sets of eight

Lower Back

Back Extensions, lift torso, feet on the floor, hold for eight counts, rest for eight counts, repeat three times

Cool-Down Stretch
Hamstring/Glute/Hip Stretch I, II, and III
Inner Thigh Stretch
Outer Thigh Stretch
Upper-Back Stretch
Lower-Back Stretch
Abdominal Stretch I, II, and III

DAY 7:
Where do you go from here? It's up to you.

THE LOVE

When the film director Steven Soderbergh won his Oscar for *Traffic* in 2000, he accepted the statuette on behalf of "anyone who spends part of their day creating." But isn't that all of us? The often grim and frustrating realities of life compel us all to create. Faith, the unwavering belief in something for which there is no proof, is a creative act we all practice every second of every day. Faith is the ultimate creative solution. And it is the final and most important principle we'll pack in our bag for our journey to holistic wellness.

Like will and desire, self-love and appreciation, activation, discipline, and emotional healing, faith needs to be implemented consciously. Faith is not a given, it's not a guarantee. It's a principle, and the ability to actively exercise it only comes after you've streamlined your mind and plugged it back into your body with the previous five principles.

Wellness doesn't happen overnight. And it's not going to happen at all if you stall, backtrack, and second-guess yourself along the way. A solid foundation of will and desire clearly and assertively stated as a simple realistic affirmation paves the way for the self-love and appreciation you need to invest in yourself. Activating *ah-hah!* overstanding and using a disciple's curiosity to inform your conscious mind encourages you to feed your body with conscious intent. Emotional healing keeps you on track away from using food as a drug. But faith in the idea of a better, healthier life for you and your family—and in turn, the whole planet—is what ties it all together.

Regardless of what religion you do or don't practice, there are certain dogmas you have learned to live by. But if believing those boilerplate unquestionable dogmas—Eve sinned, God is love, God is vengeance, God is dead, all life is suffering, Allah, Jesus, or Jehovah says this, that, or the other—doesn't unite your inner and outer self and connect you with those around you, they're not articles of faith at all. No offense to anybody's anything, but a holistic wellness lifestyle won't take if you confuse faith with dogma. Without conscious, creative, applied faith behind it, dogmatic belief becomes a blanket to pull up over your head and hide under. Dogma is a cop-out, but you're not going to get well by giving up. Dogma is a eulogy written on a tombstone, but you can't get on the road to wellness by starting at the end. Dogma invites unconsciousness. Dream all you want along the way, but be conscious of the steps you're taking.

Dogma disconnects. Faith is a flashlight on the road ahead. It requires you to be conscious and to reinvest in the other five principles. Faith connects. Faith flows. Faith lets you love and be loved.

My Creole-speaking Sistahs and Brothers from the Caribbean use the word *faire* interchangeably to mean both "to make" and "to do." They say that experience is the best teacher, and you've just spent five weeks acquiring invaluable experience that will help you make or do anything that your heart wills and desires in the future. What else is left to do? The rest of your life.

All it takes in the end is faith—faith in yourself and your cells, faith in the informed yet instinctive choices you make in order to be well, and, most important, faith in the love that comes down around us when we're living the best way we can live. The practices of both doing and making are the same when it comes to love. Everything you do is an act of love built on faith. Everything you make has love's strength and faith's intentions built into it. It would be a terrible waste of all the work you've put into

The Remedy not to share the love that resulted when faith allowed you to cleanse and unify and revive and restore the flow.

No man is an island. No woman walks truly alone. An integral part of holistic health and wellness is exercising the strength, sensitivity, energy, and renewed ability to connect with others that are the gifts of a unified body and mind. The mate that you choose can be part of your Remedy, or they can be part of your problem. The choice is up to you. I advise my Sistahs and my Brothers to seek out a partner who is mentally, spiritually, and yes, physically conscious. A mate that is willing to reach out and heal herself, her family, and her community. Your woman or man should be a healer. She or he needs to be willing to restore your soul and rejuvenate your spirit. She or he should give you energy to come alive again and again. You mate is your friend, your lover, your comforter, your sanctuary. Love is sacred, so your mate is sacred.

I'll leave you with this poem:

If making love is formulating
and formulating is creating,
can one
make,
create,
or formulate love
by simply having sex?
makingLOVE is building foundations so sex is never the center of our
    circle,
but rather rays of illumination like that of the sun,
you enhance the beauty of my light.
makingLOVE is sitting at the park reading Skekum, Fanon, and Ani,
    building and exchanging energies.
makingLOVE is eating dinner with the family as you glide your hand
    between my legs going unnoticed by anyone. Then later sucking on my
    neck as I wash the dishes and you dry.
makingLOVE is feeding babies in the middle of the night.

makingLOVE is sitting in bed reading nighttime stories to the children. makingLOVE is working together, cleansing together and sharing responsibilities.

makingLOVE is sitting in the hospital at 3.a.m. falling asleep on your shoulder as you hold Mama's hand 'round midnight and we wait for the doctor to return with a diagnosis.

makingLOVE is making decisions together and honoring them.

makingLOVE is when I bite my tongue and let you discipline our boy so he can grow up to be in your image, a good man.

makingLOVE is running a business and a family together. makingLOVE is cherishing the partnerships that we have created and holding them sacred.

makingLOVE is learning together, building the future together and staying aligned.

makingLOVE is not just listening when your lover speaks, but learning so you may grow as one breath.

makingLOVE is not always agreeing; but it is acknowledging individuality and respecting difference.

makingLOVE is apologizing when you know you're wrong and remaining objective when you think you're right.

makingLOVE is having patience when situations are not as you would like, and having foresight to progress destinies.

makingLOVE is teaching and leading by example.

makingLOVE is when you nurse my battered wings and anoint my broken spirit keeping me warmly nurtured in your grace until I am healthy enough to take flight again.

makingLOVE is praying together and meditating together so we may achieve a better relationship with our inner selves, nature and the universe.

makingLOVE is walking in the rain as Aset's purifier purges our souls and grows our flowers.

makingLOVE is not jumping to conclusions, but giving the benefit of the doubt.

makingLOVE is the sore soldier eyes of Gil Scott-Heron being kissed by the soft succulent affection of Sarah Vaughn and then re-energized with the charisma of Sweet Honey in the Rock.

makingLOVE is not playing games or trickery. makingLOVE is being straight up and straightforward.

makingLOVE is looking through another, finding weaknesses, and building them up, finding strengths, and magnifying them.

makingLOVE is not "I told you so," nor is it blame, guilt, or shame.

makingLOVE is cultivation without suffocation or humiliation.

makingLOVE is positive reinforcement.

makingLOVE is freedom, not control.

makingLOVE is not prejudgment or persecution. makingLOVE is pursuing preservation.

makingLOVE is supporting each other's experimentation even when you are unsure of the conclusions. Sometimes, makingLOVE is letting me fall.

makingLOVE is countless years of support and love and fights and tears and forgiveness. makingLOVE is learning how to rejuvenate and restore.

makingLOVE is when you came inside of me and together we conceived life.

makingLOVE is building nations.

Salute!
Supa Nova Slom

seven

Recipes

Supa Mega Greens

1 tsp. spirulina
1 tsp. sun chlorella
1 tsp. powdered wheatgrass (or 3 oz. of fresh wheatgrass juice)
1 tsp. powdered alfalfa grass (or 3 oz. juiced fresh alfalfa grass)
1 tsp. powdered green barley grass (or 3 oz. fresh Green Barley grass juice)
½ tsp. fresh ginger, juiced (two or three decent-sized fingers of fresh ginger)
1 cup dandelion greens, juiced or powdered

Mix ingredients in a separate container, then add to juice or gallon jug of water.

My Supa Mega Greens powder combines low-temperature dehydrated, highly concentrated forms of these fresh juices and greens and is available from www.supanovaslom.com.

Chickpea Soup with Okra and Scallions (vegan)

4 cloves crushed garlic
1 medium onion, chopped

¼ cup cold-pressed virgin olive oil
1 large or two medium tomatoes, skinned and diced
1 cup sliced okra
1 dash of cider vinegar
1 pinch cayenne pepper
Pinch cinnamon
2½ cups dried chickpeas, soaked and drained, or canned chickpeas,
    thoroughly rinsed
2 cups vegetable stock
3 scallions, sliced thin
Black pepper

Sauté garlic and onion in olive oil in a soup pot and combine with tomatoes, okra, scallions, vinegar, and spices. Simmer covered at low heat until okra is cooked through and tender (about 15 minutes).

Add chickpeas and vegetable stock. If mixture level doesn't cover chickpeas, add more stock. If mixture is too thin, add more chickpeas. Cover and simmer for 30 minutes or until chickpeas are tender but not mushy. Remove from heat, serve, and garnish with scallions and black pepper to taste. Serves 4 to 6.

Oven-Steamed Fish

¼ tsp. celery salt
¼ tsp. garlic powder
¼ tsp. paprika
1 Tbsp. cold-pressed olive oil
1 4 oz. fish filet, lean
½ green pepper
1 red onion

Mix celery salt, garlic powder, paprika, and olive oil together in a small bowl. Place fish filet in a glass baking dish and spoon mixture over filet to cover; refrigerate overnight. Drain excess; marinate the following day.

Preheat oven to 325°. Dice green pepper and onion and add to dish. Bake for 15 to 20 minutes, or until fish is cooked through and flaky. Serves 1.

Kidney Bean, Okra, and Tomato Stew (vegan)

2 to 3 Tbsp. cold-pressed virgin olive oil
4 to 6 cloves of garlic, crushed
1 large red onion, chopped
½ cup chopped celery
½ cup chopped okra
1 cup chopped carrots
Dash of sage
1 tsp. oregano
Dash of thyme
½ tsp. rosemary
4 tomatoes, skinned and diced
2 to 3 Tbsp. Bragg's Liquid Aminos
⅔ cup uncooked brown rice or wild rice
2 to 3 cups water
2 cups dried kidney beans, soaked and cooked, or canned kidney beans,
    thoroughly rinsed
Black pepper
¼ cup cilantro, chopped

Heat oil in a large soup pot. Sauté garlic, onion, celery, okra, and
carrots with sage, oregano, thyme, and rosemary until onion is clear
and okra, celery, and carrots are slightly tender. Stir in tomatoes,
Bragg's, rice, and water and bring to a boil. Reduce heat, cover, and
simmer for 45 minutes, adding water if needed to keep the rice moist.

Stir in beans and simmer on low heat for another 10 to 15 minutes,
until beans and rice are both tender. Garnish with cilantro. Serves 6 to 8.

Curry Mock Chicken Salad on Salad Greens (vegan)

¼ cup sunflower seeds
½ cup cashews
½ cup pecans
½ medium cucumber, chopped
1 red onion, chopped
1 carrot, chopped
Pinch of curry powder

Juice of ½ lemon
1 tub (about 7 oz.) Suneen or other brand veggie "chicken" salad
or
8 oz. medium-chunk TVP, soaked and drained, lightly braised, mixed with
    2 Tbsp. vegan mayonnaise and ¼ cup celery, chopped
Vegan mayonnaise
½ cup arugula
½ head iceberg lettuce

In a mixing bowl, combine seeds, nuts, cucumber, onion, carrot, curry powder, lemon juice, "chicken" salad or TVP mix, and additional mayo (between ½ to 1½ Tbsp. depending on how rich you like it). Serve on bed of lettuce and garnish with arugula and lettuce to taste. Serves 2 to 4.

"Beef" TVP Stew Beans (vegan)

2 cups TVP
¼ cup red wine
3¾ cups vegetable broth
2 Tbsp. cold-pressed virgin olive oil
4 to 6 garlic cloves, crushed
1 large bell pepper, chopped
1 large onion, chopped
2 Tbsp. fresh ginger, crushed, with juice
2 tsp. cayenne pepper
1½ tsp. oregano
2 medium sweet potatoes (or summer or winter squash), peeled and
    chopped into chunks
1 cup dried black-eyed peas, soaked and drained, or canned black-eyed
    peas rinsed

Soak TVP in wine and 1¾ cups vegetable broth overnight.

In a soup pot, heat olive oil and sauté garlic, bell pepper, and onion, adding ginger, cayenne pepper, and oregano before onion mixture browns. Add sweet potato chunks and remaining broth and bring to a boil. Reduce heat, cover, and simmer for 10 to 15 minutes or until sweet potatoes are tender. Add black-eyed peas. Drain TVP, then stir it into the pot. Cover and simmer for another 10 to 15 minutes.

Serve over brown rice or with sprouted wheat bread. Serves 4 to 6.

"Beef" TVP/Soya Protein (vegan)

1 lb. TVP chunks, soaked
4 Tbsp. cold-pressed virgin olive oil
1 cup chopped red onions
½ tsp. garlic powder
1 cup chopped green bell peppers
½ tsp. celery salt
1 tsp. sage
½ tsp. cumin
2 cups distilled water

Prepare TVP by soaking it in about 2 pints of water (1:1 ratio of TVP to water) for 20 minutes; drain. For extra flavor, marinate the soaked and drained TVP in a half cup of wine.

In a skillet, heat 2 Tbsp. olive oil and sauté onions, garlic, and peppers. Add celery salt, sage, and cumin. Add TVP and cook until browned. Reduce heat, add water and remaining olive oil, and let the mixture simmer for 15 minutes. Serves 3 to 5.

Blueberry Buckwheat Pancakes (vegan)

1 cup buckwheat flour (or ½ cup each of buckwheat and unbleached
    whole-wheat flour)
¾ tsp. baking powder
Pinch of baking soda
1 cup soy, almond, or rice milk
1 tsp. stevia
1 tsp. vanilla
2 to 3 Tbsp. chopped pecans, walnuts, or almonds, if desired
1 pint blueberries, fresh or frozen

Blend flour, baking powder, and baking soda thoroughly in a mixing bowl. Add milk, stevia, and vanilla and continue to mix until the batter is free of clumps. Stir in nuts and gently stir in blueberries before spooning out onto a preheated frying pan or griddle that has been prepared with cooking spray. As pancakes begin to bubble, sprinkle additional blueberries onto the wet batter facing up.

Once thoroughly bubbled, flip and allow to brown on the other side. The amount of bubbling will depend on skillet temp, thickness of batter, and the amount of fruit and nuts, so use the results of the first pancake as a guide of doneness. Yields 8–10 pancakes.

Chef Ali's Home Style Signature BBQ Tofu (vegan)

Inspired by my grandmother's BBQ chicken.

1 block extra-firm tofu*
2 Tbsp. parsley
1 Tbsp. sea salt
2 Tbsp. garlic powder
1 Tbsp. cumin
1 Tbsp. dill
2 cups whole wheat flour (nongluten substitutes include brown rice flour, quinoa flour, or buckwheat flour)
1 cup cold-pressed virgin olive oil

Slice tofu into 1-inch strips the long way and then cut those in half.

Place parsley, salt, garlic powder, cumin, dill, and flour in a ziplock bag and shake well. Add tofu and shake until well coated.

In a skillet, heat olive oil and sauté coated tofu strips for about 5 minutes, turning as needed, until both sides are golden brown. Place the browned strips on a paper towel to drain excess oil, and cool.

Preheat the oven to 325°. Place the tofu in a baking pan and coat with Chef Ali's BBQ sauce (recipe below). Bake for 20 mintues. Serves 4.

* For an even firmer consistency, wrap the sliced, uncooked tofu in paper towel and gently press excess water out of it. Place the drained tofu in the freezer overnight. Thaw completely the following day, then continue.

Chef Ali's BBQ Sauce (vegan)

16 oz. can organic tomato sauce
1 cup blackstrap molasses
2 Tbsp. chili pepper
½ cup lemon juice, freshly squeezed

6 tsp. stevia
3 Tbsp. garlic powder
1 Tbsp. bee pollen
2 Tbsp. Italian seasoning

Mix all ingredients in a bowl, pour into a jar, and refrigerate. Equivalent to a 20 oz. bottle of barbecue sauce.

Baked Tofu Spinach Couscous (vegan)

2½ Tbsp. cold-pressed virgin olive oil
4 to 6 cloves garlic, crushed
1 large red onion
½ to 1 tsp. cumin
1 medium bag baby spinach
1 large block extra-firm tofu, drained, frozen, and thawed
1 box organic couscous
1 cup vegetable stock

Heat olive oil in a saucepan and sauté garlic and onion with cumin until clarified. Add spinach and continue cooking until spinach has wilted. Crumble tofu into spinach mixture and continue to sauté until tofu begins to brown.

Preheat oven to 350°. Spoon tofu mixture into a baking dish. Cover with foil and bake for 15 to 20 minutes.

Follow package instructions for preparing couscous on stovetop, substituting a cup of vegetable stock for the equivalent amount of water in the recipe, and cook until fluffy.

Remove foil from tofu and put baking dish under broiler for 3 to 5 minutes until tofu is browned, being careful not to burn.

Serve couscous topped with tofu spinach crumble. Serves 3 to 5.

Vegan Corn Bread (vegan)

2 cups soy, rice, or almond milk
2 tsp. apple cider vinegar
2 cups organic cornmeal
1 cup whole-wheat flour

2 tsp. baking powder
½ tsp. sea salt
⅓ cup canola oil
⅓ cup applesauce, unsweetened
¼ cup husked sweet corn kernels or thawed frozen corn kernels
2 Tbsp. maple syrup

Preheat oven to 400°. Spray the inside of a 9×13 baking pan with nonstick cooking spray.

Whisk milk and vinegar together in a bowl and set aside. Combine cornmeal, flour, baking powder, and salt in a large bowl. Add oil, applesauce, corn kernels, and maple syrup to the milk mixture and whisk until frothy. Combine wet and dry ingredients until thoroughly mixed. Spoon batter into baking pan. Bake 30 minutes, checking to see that top of bread browns slightly and that a toothpick inserted into the center of the bread comes out clean. Serves 3 to 4.

Garden Greens (raw/vegan)

1 cup basil, fresh chopped
½ cup green pepper, chopped
½ cup kale, chopped
½ cup spinach, chopped
1 cup fresh mint, chopped
1½ tsp. sea salt
½ cup arugula, chopped
½ cup watercress, chopped
½ cup cucumber, chopped
½ cup string beans, diced
¼ cup cold-pressed virgin olive oil
½ cup lemon juice, freshly squeezed
½ cup broccoli, chopped
½ cup chickweed, chopped

Combine all of the ingredients in a large salad bowl, mix well, and serve. Serves about 4.

Chickpeas, Zucchini, Mushrooms, and Sun-dried Tomatoes over Pasta (vegan)

3 Tbsp. cold-pressed virgin olive oil
2 to 4 cloves of garlic, crushed
1 onion, chopped
Large pinch of oregano
1 cup sliced mushrooms
1 large zucchini, sliced
1 box (8 oz.) whole-wheat, corn, buckwheat, or Jerusalem artichoke pasta
1 large can or one heaping cup chickpeas, soaked and cooked
1 cup sun-dried tomatoes
Black pepper to taste

Sauté garlic and onion in saucepan. Add oregano, mushrooms, and zucchini and cook until zucchini and mushrooms become tender.

Using a separate pot, follow package instructions for pasta. While pasta is cooking, add chickpeas and tomatoes to the vegetable mix and stir. Cover, reduce heat, and simmer 6 to 10 minutes. Drain pasta, place in bowls, and spoon veggies on top. Serves 3 to 5.

Pan-Cooked Broccoli Jump Off (vegan)

1 large head broccoli
1 medium onion, diced
1 medium green or red pepper, chopped
1 cup cold-pressed virgin olive oil
1 Tbsp. garlic powder
1 tsp. sea salt
1 tsp. Bragg's Liquid Aminos
1 Tbsp. sage
1 tsp. cilantro
1 tsp. chili powder

Trim off broccoli stems and break up individual florets. Combine all other ingredients in mixing bowl, add broccoli, cover, and set aside for an hour to marinate.

Preheat oven to 350°. Pour marinated broccoli into a baking dish, cover with foil, and bake for 30 to 35 minutes (broccoli should still be tender). Remove foil and place under broiler for 3 to 5 minutes. Let cool before serving. Serves 4.

Green Lentil Vegiole Soup (vegan)

2 Tbsp. olive oil
2 garlic cloves, crushed
1 large onion, chopped
2 carrots, sliced
Ground pepper to taste
2 large tomatoes, diced
1 cup dry green lentils
1 quart vegetable broth or stock
1 pinch of dried thyme
Juice of ½ lemon
2 bay leaves
¾ cup whole-wheat, spinach, or Jerusalem artichoke macaroni.

Heat olive oil in a soup pot and sauté garlic, onion, and carrots with black pepper until vegetables are cooked, but not browned. Add tomatoes and stir in lentils until they are well coated. Stir in vegetable stock, thyme, and lemon juice. Bring to a boil, then reduce heat. Add bay leaves and simmer covered about 30 to 40 minutes.

Stir in macaroni and simmer on low heat, cooking for 8 to 10 minutes stirring occasionally, until pasta is al dente.

Veggie Cole Slaw (vegan)

1 large head of cabbage, chopped fine or julienned
1 cup grated carrot
1 cup chopped bell pepper
½ cup chopped radish
½ cup chopped jicama
1 finger of ginger peeled and finely chopped
1 medium onion, diced
Dollop of veggie mayonnaise, to taste

Combine all vegetable ingredients. Add ½ cup Chef Ali's Home-made Dressing (recipe below) and veggie mayonnaise and either mix in a bowl or shake up in a jar. For creamier slaw, add more mayo; for tangier, use less.

Chef Ali's Homemade Dressing (vegan)

3 Tbsp. organic apple cider vinegar
1 tsp. sea salt
Pinch of cayenne pepper
½ tsp. chopped ginger
¼ cup cold-pressed virgin olive oil
Juice of ½ lime

Combine all ingredients in a small bowl. Pour into a jar, seal, and refrigerate for use.

Cauliflower Power Dip (vegan/raw)

3½ cups cauliflower
2 cups raw cashews
Juice of 1 lemon
3 to 4 cloves garlic, chopped
1 Tbsp. sea salt
1 Tbsp. dill, fresh chopped

Blend cauliflower in blender or food processor until finely chopped. Add remaining ingredients, blend until smooth, and serve with toasted pita. Serves 3 to 5.

Live Spiced Rice (vegan/raw)

½ cup green peppers, chopped
½ cup yellow bell peppers, chopped
½ cup red bell peppers, chopped
½ cup purple onions, chopped
½ cup red beets, diced
½ cup green peas

½ cup purple cabbage, chopped and diced
1 cup raw almonds, chopped
1 cup sprouted brown rice
2 pinches cayenne pepper
3 to 5 cloves garlic, crushed
1 Tbsp. ginger, minced
Juice of ½ lemon
2 Tbsp. of organic apple cider vinegar

This one's all in the prep. Once you're done chopping, just mix all the ingredients in a large bowl, place the mixture in a dish, serve, and enjoy! Serves 2.

Carrot "Tuna" (vegan)

5 large or 10 small carrots
½ cup celery
½ cup chopped green bell pepper
2 to 3 cloves garlic, chopped
½ cup nori seaweed
1 Tbsp. parsley
1 tsp. sea salt
¼ tsp. paprika
1 cup vegan mayonnaise
¼ cup olive oil
2 cups alfalfa sprouts

Juice the carrots and set the juice aside. Remove the carrot pulp from juicer and place in a mixing bowl. Add celery, pepper, garlic, seaweed, parsley, sea salt, and paprika. Stirring gently, add mayonnaise and olive oil.

Serve garnished with alfalfa sprouts on a bed of greens, or in a pita. Serves 3 to 5.

Blueberry Oat Muffins (vegan)

2 cups distilled water
1 cup raw rolled oats
1 cup sesame butter

1 cup agave nectar
4 tsp. egg substitute
4 cups almond milk
4 cups whole-wheat flour (nongluten substitutes include brown rice
    flour, quinoa flour, or buckwheat flour)
5 tsp. organic baking soda
1½ tsp. sea salt
2 cups blueberries

Preheat oven to 375°. Mix water and oats in mixing bowl and set aside.

In a separate bowl, mix sesame butter, agave, and egg substitute. Add almond milk, flour, baking soda, and sea salt and mix well. Stir in soaked oats. Gently fold in blueberries.

Prepare muffin pan with olive oil and a light dusting of flour. Spoon in the batter and bake for 15 to 20 minutes. Makes 12 muffins.

Veggie Wrap (vegan/raw)

2 Tbsp. pitted black olives, chopped
1 cup portobello mushrooms, chopped
1 cup green bell peppers, diced
1 cup green scallions, chopped
¼ cup cucumber, diced
2 carrots, diced
½ cup olive oil
Juice of 1 lemon
1 medium tomato, diced
1 tsp. sea salt
1 Tbsp. fresh oregano, chopped
1 Tbsp. fresh rosemary, chopped
6 large Romaine lettuce leaves

Combine all ingredients except lettuce leaves in a bowl and mix well. Spoon out mixture and spread onto lettuce leaves. Roll each leaf closed, serve, and enjoy. Serves 3 (2 wraps each).

Bulgur Wheat (vegan)

1 cup bulgur wheat
1 cup warm water
2 ripe avocados, pitted and cubed
½ cup diced red bell peppers
1 cup diced cucumber
1 Tbsp. minced garlic
1 cup chopped fresh mint
⅓ cup cold-pressed virgin olive oil
Juice of ½ lime
½ tsp. sea salt

Soak bulgur in a bowl with warm water for 5 to 7 minutes and drain.

Combine remaining ingredients, add bulgur, and mix thoroughly. Serves 3.

Broccoli Hype (vegan/raw)

2 bunches of broccoli
1 medium red onion, chopped
½ cup red pepper
2½ chopped cups green pepper
½ cup chopped yellow pepper
1 Tbsp. fresh sage
1 Tbsp. oregano
1 Tbsp. minced garlic
1 Tbsp. fresh lemon thyme

Combine all ingredients in a large mixing bowl. Pour into a serving dish and top with Chef Ali's Homemade Dressing (*see page* 199 *for recipe*). Serves 2 to 3.

Kidney Cleanser Supa Juice (16 oz. glass)

1 bunch of parsley
½ cucumber
1 bunch of watercress

Liver Cleanser Supa Juice (16 oz. glass)

1 stalk of broccoli
2 stalks of kale
1 stalk of chard

Blood Builder Supa Juice (16 oz. glass)

1 cucumber
1 handful of spinach
1 handful of parsley
1 stalk of celery
2 stalks of kale
½ beet

Lymphatic Flush Supa Juice (16 oz. glass)

¼ stalk of ginger
1 bunch of parsley
1 piece of fresh garlic
2 medium-sized carrots
1 stalk of celery

Respiratory Cleanser Supa Juice (16 oz. glass)

2 radishes
1 scallion
1 bunch of parsley
2 cucumbers

Immune Booster Supa Juice (16 oz. glass)

8 oz. cup fresh cranberries
3 apples
¼ stalk of ginger

Colon Cleanser Supa Juice (16 oz. glass)

1 Tbsp flaxseed oil
2 stalks of celery
1 stalk of broccoli
3 stalks of kale
1 bunch of fresh fennel
2 carrots

Acknowledgments

Now y'all know there's an endless list of you out there all around the globe and cosmos that deserve acknowledgments, praise, and thanks. So if you feel that you have in any way contributed to the success, the shaping, the molding, and the manifestation of this project and move-ment or the overall Supa Nova brand, please write your name here: _____.

I would also like to extend acknowledgments to the Creator of us all; my family; countless friends; and *The Remedy* team: Ali, Queen, Haqq, Damon, Shawn, Bruce, Mary Ellen, and Matthew. Also to those seen and unseen, and humanity's unlimited potential to be the change that we truly seek.

Your guide on this wellness journey,
Supa Nova Slom
The Medicine Man

About the Author

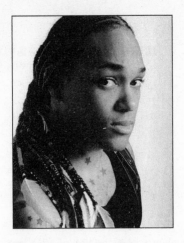

A second-generation vegetarian from a family of health activists, Supa Nova Slom is the living embodiment of the wellness lifestyle, and living proof that the principles of The Remedy work. Known in hip-hop circles and on the streets of Crown Heights, Brooklyn, as the Medicine Man, Supa Nova is a wellness counselor to hip-hop's elite, a tireless advocate and educator about diet and health on behalf of Brooklyn's youth, and an accomplished rapper in his own right.

In addition to devoting nearly half of his life to working with young people on health and empowerment issues through the Hip-Hop Meditation Cipher, Supa Nova created and produced the documentary film *Holistic Wellness for the Hip-Hop Generation,* featuring Eryka Badu, Common, and Ben Vereen. He is a frequent cohost on Chuck D's show on Power 105.1 in New York City, and has delivered his message of wellness and nutrition on Air America radio; WBAI, KISS FM, and WBLS in New York; and KJLH in Los Angeles. He has also been profiled in *The Source, Undercover,* and *Billboard,* and on Allhiphop.com and BET.com.

More information about The Remedy and Supa Nova can be found at www.supanovaslom.com.